Gestational Diabetes Mellitus - An Overview with Some Recent Advances

Edited by Amita Ray

Published in London, United Kingdom

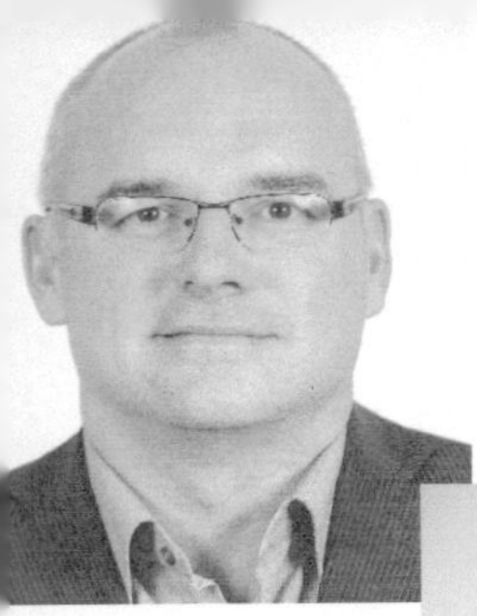

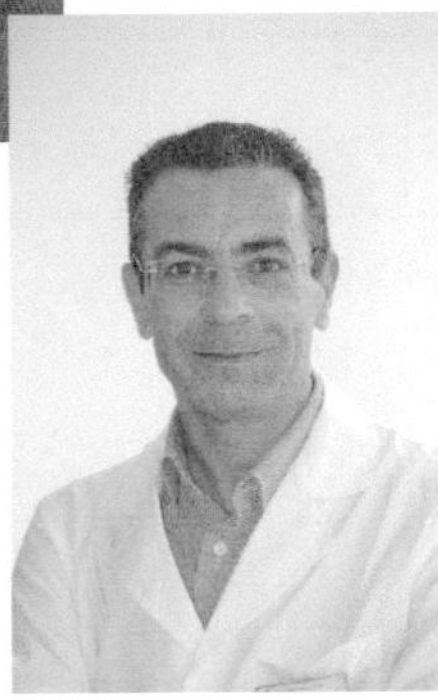

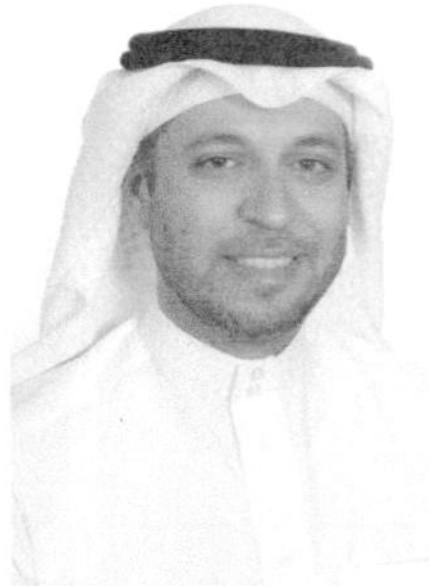

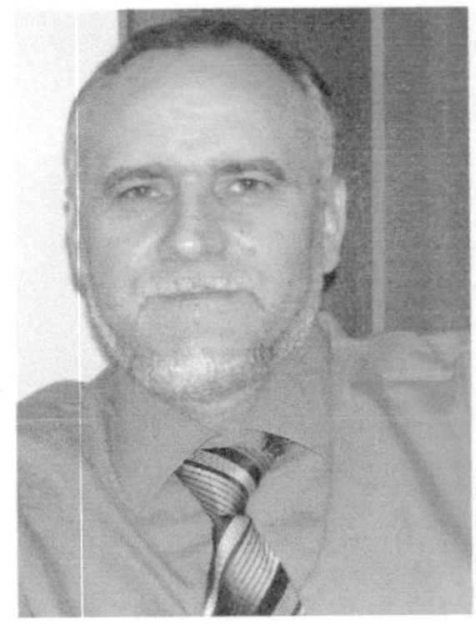

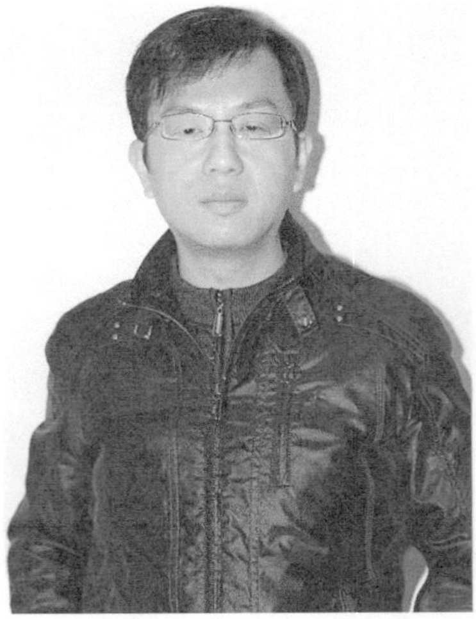

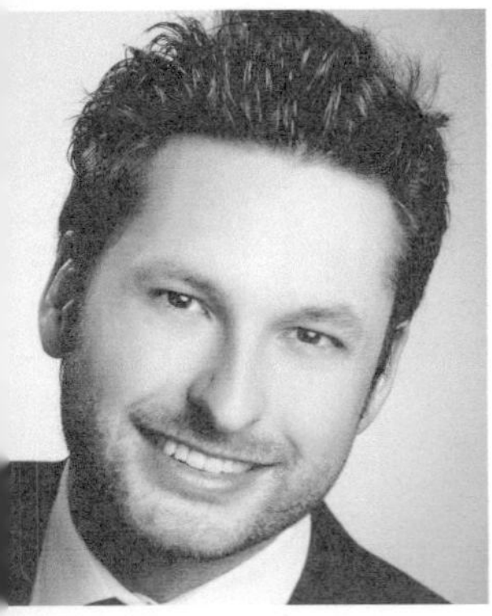

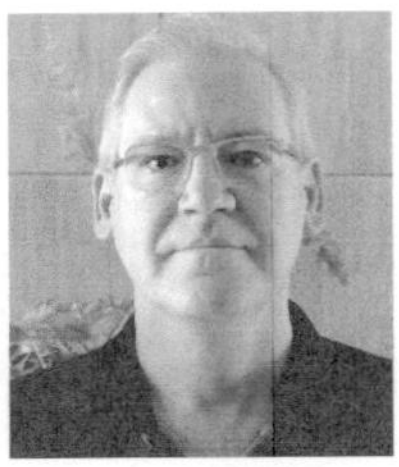

IntechOpen

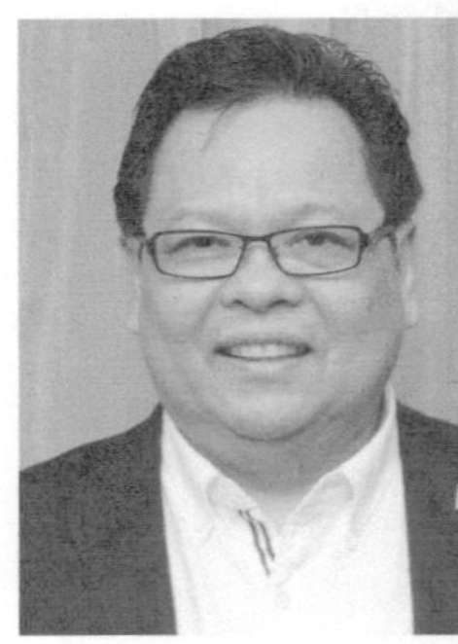

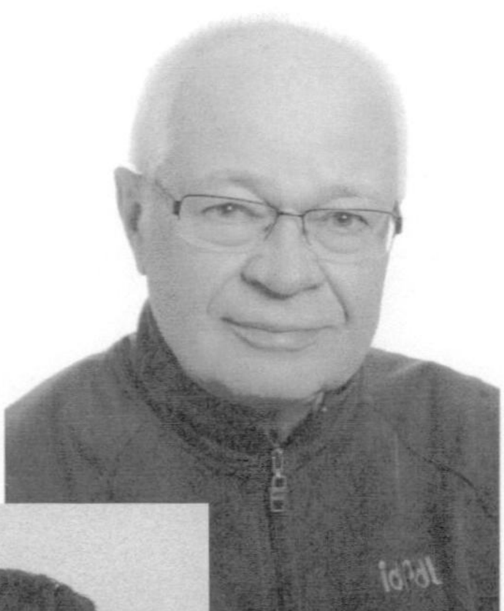

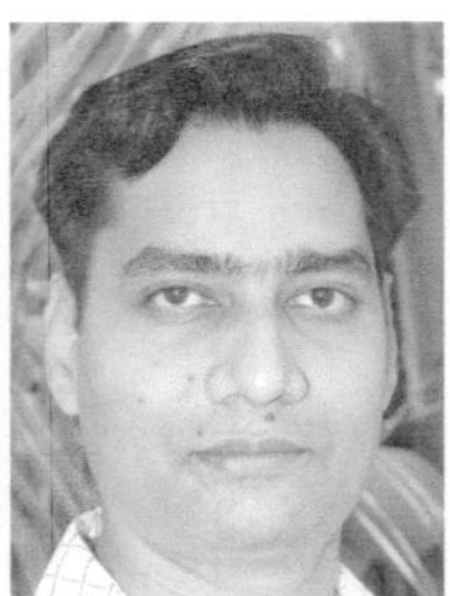

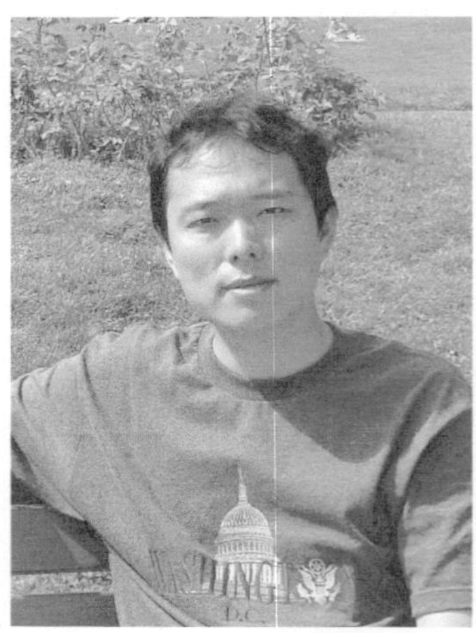

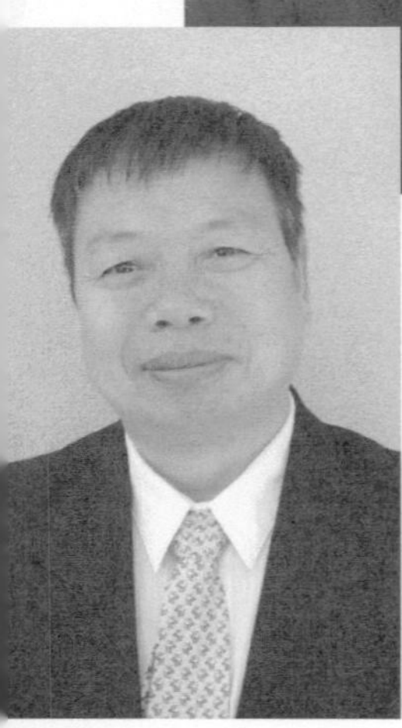

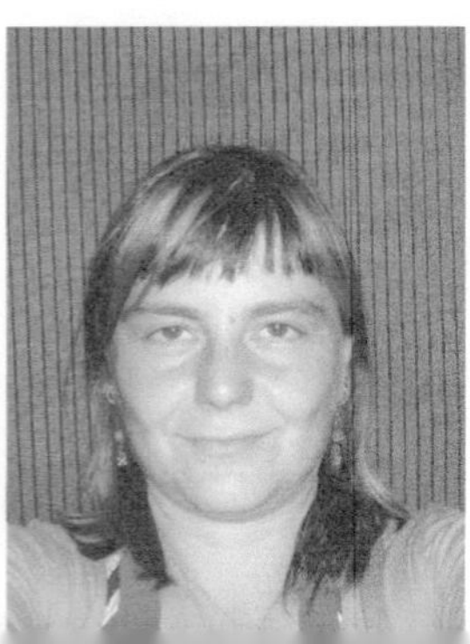

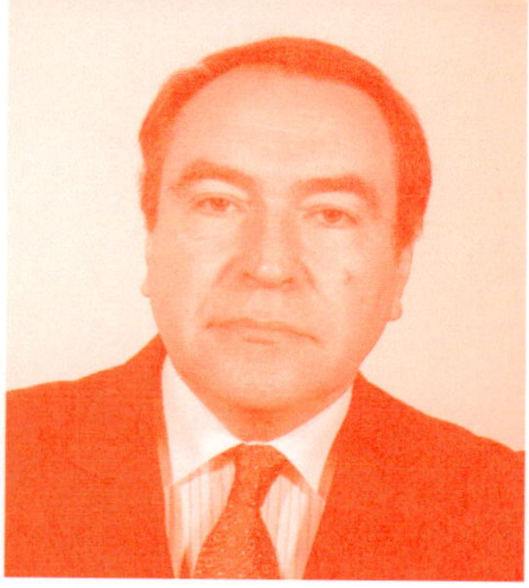

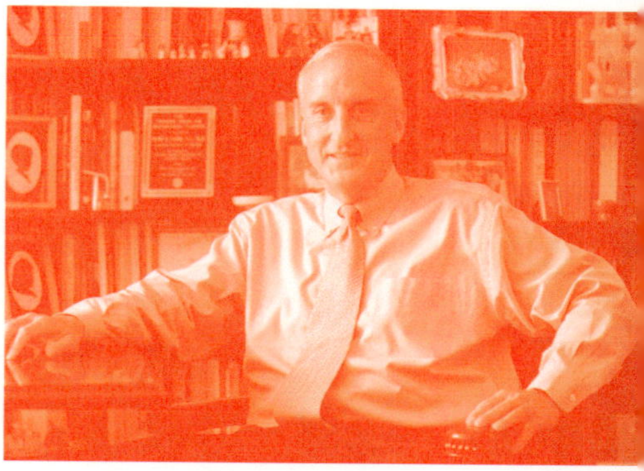

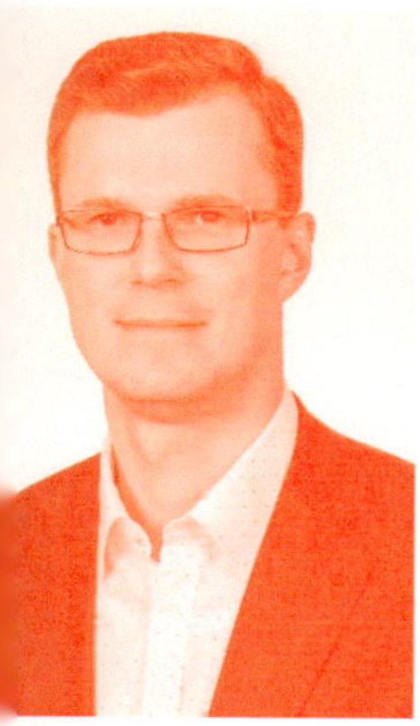

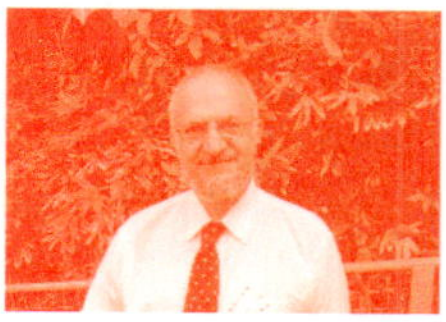

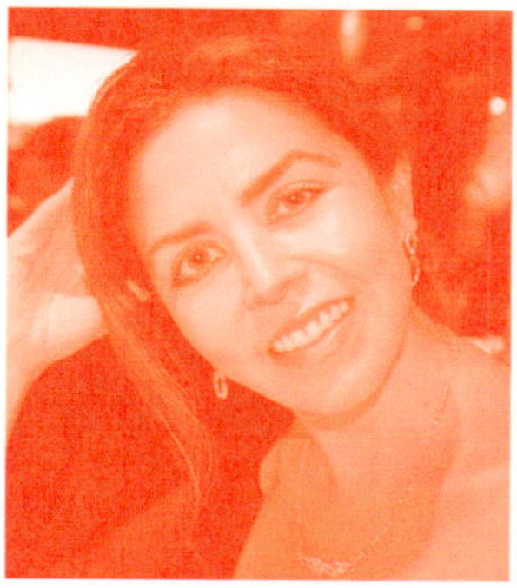

Supporting open minds since 2005

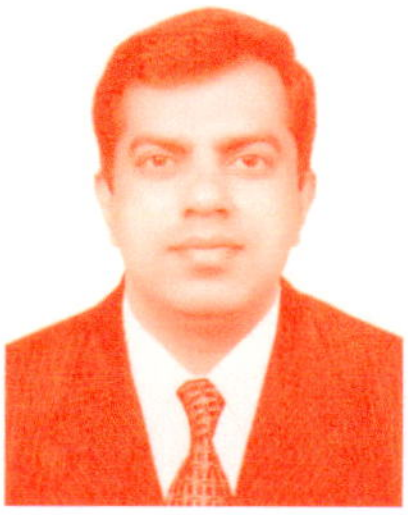

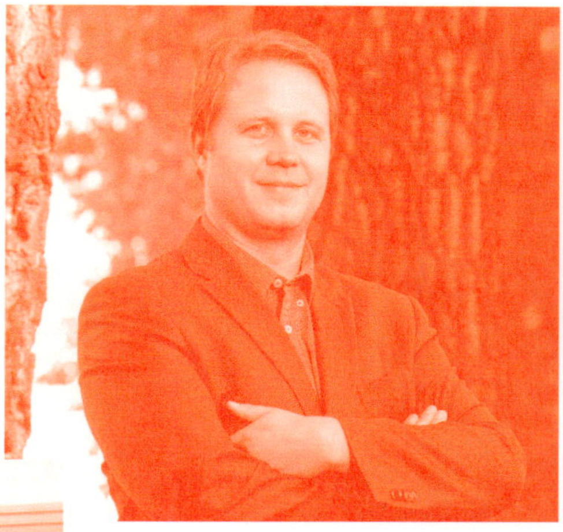

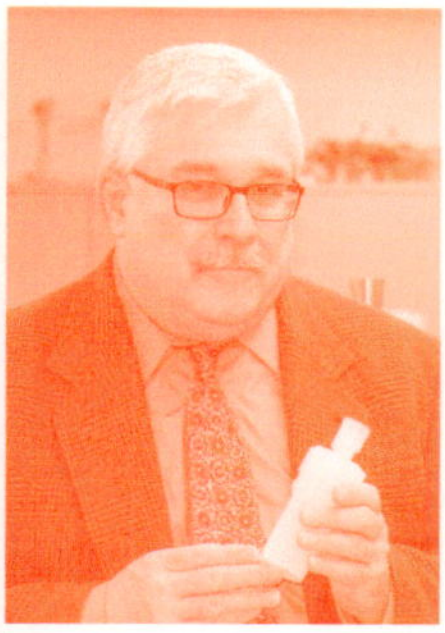

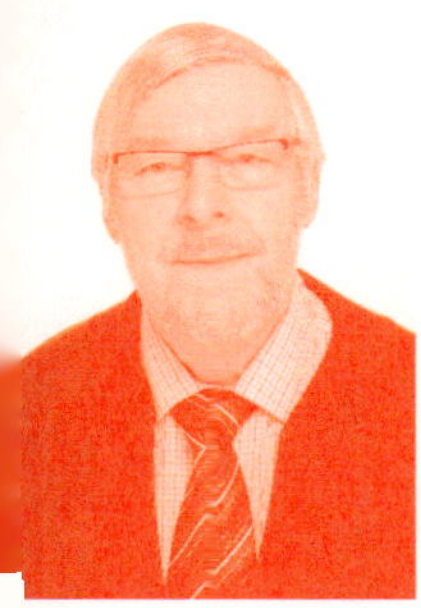

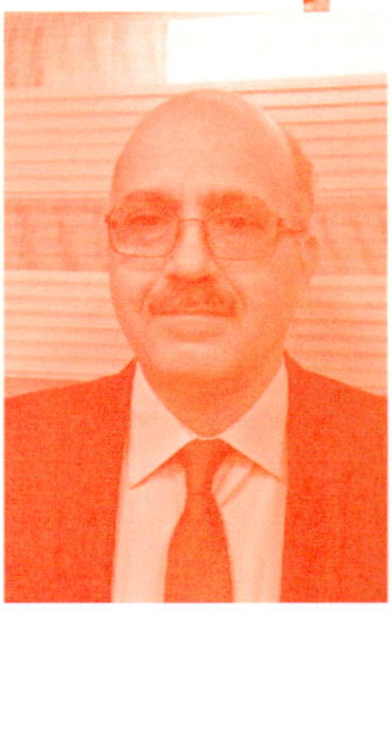

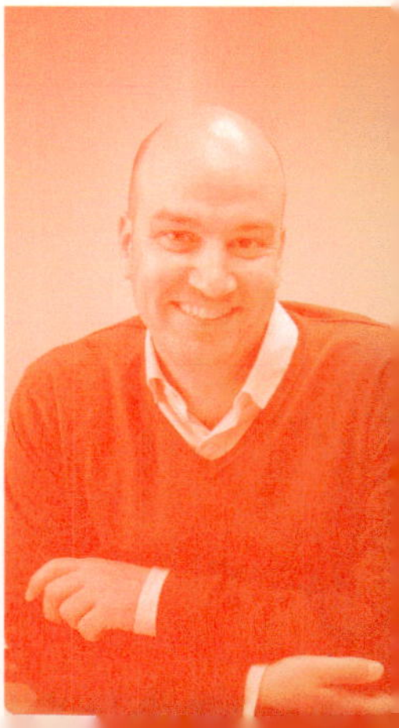

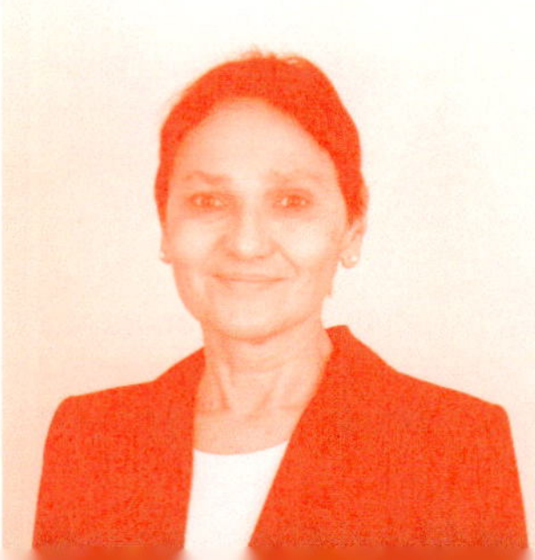

Gestational Diabetes Mellitus - An Overview with Some Recent Advances
http://dx.doi.org/10.5772/intechopen.73941
Edited by Amita Ray

Contributors
Ahmed Maged, Renata Saucedo, Jorge Valencia, Maria Isabel Peña-Cano, Enrique Morales-Avila, Arturo Zarate, Carmen Pheiffer, Sumaiya Adam, Stephanie Dias, Paul Rheeder, Anca Pantea Stoian, Roxana Adriana Stoica, Simona Diana Stefan, Víctor Sánchez-Margalet, Pilar Guadix, Antonio Pérez-Pérez, Teresa Vilariño-García, José L. Dueñas, Julieta Maymó, Cecilia Varone, Arshiya Shamim, Tarique Mahmood, Paramdeep Bagga, Farogh Ahsan, Mohd Haris Siddiqui, Hh Siddiqui, Amita Ray

First published in London, United Kingdom, 2020 by IntechOpen
IntechOpen is the global imprint of INTECHOPEN LIMITED, registered in England and Wales, registration number: 11086078, 7th floor, 10 Lower Thames Street, London, EC3R 6AF, United Kingdom
Printed in Croatia

British Library Cataloguing-in-Publication Data
A catalogue record for this book is available from the British Library

Additional hard and PDF copies can be obtained from orders@intechopen.com

Gestational Diabetes Mellitus - An Overview with Some Recent Advances
Edited by Amita Ray
p. cm.
Print ISBN 978-1-78984-733-8
Online ISBN 978-1-78985-187-8
eBook (PDF) ISBN 978-1-78985-188-5

For EU product safety concerns:
IN TECH d.o.o., Prolaz Marije Krucifikse Kozulić 3, 51000 Rijeka, Croatia, info@intechopen.com or visit our website at intechopen.com.

Meet the editor

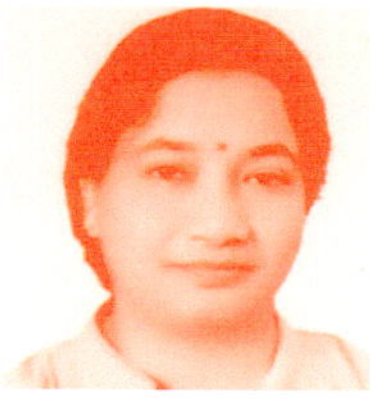

Prof. Dr. Amita Ray MBBS, MS, Obstetrics and Gynecology
Fellow Gynecology and Gynae-Oncology Royal Adelaide Hospital, South Australia
Fellow High Risk Pregnancy Management Royal Oman Hospital, Sultan Quaboos University, Oman
FAIMER Fellow (Foundation for Advancement of Medical Education and Research)
MSc MHPE (Masters in Health Professional Education)
She has worked as a clinician and medical teacher in various medical colleges all over India for the past 30 years. She is passionate about clinical work among underprivileged women with high risk complications in tribal and rural areas and equally passionate about medical education. She has introduced several innovative projects in health education, which have improved medical teacher efficiency in resource-constrained settings as a part of her FAIMER Fellowship. She has guided several post-graduate dissertations. She has several publications in reputed national and international journals including British, American, and South Asian journals of obstetrics and gynecology. She has authored and co-authored several book chapters in obstetrics and gynecology text books used as a part of undergraduate and post-graduate education in India.
Besides this, she is passionate about evidence-based medicine. She is a member of different Cochrane Groups and has authored and co-authored several Cochrane Reviews for the Cochrane Pregnancy and Childbirth Group, Cochrane Cystic Fibrosis Group, and Cochrane Infectious Diseases Group.
She is currently working as Professor and Head of the Department of Obstetrics and Gynecology at IQ City Medical College, Durgapur, West Bengal, India.

Contents

Preface

This book on gestational diabetes does not claim to cover all aspects of this complex and ever-evolving medical condition. It is an attempt by the group of authors to provide an overview, highlight important features, and bring to light certain recent advances in the diagnosis, screening, and understanding of gestational diabetes mellitus. As the book provides an overview of the condition, we are sure that reading it would provide medical undergraduates and postgraduates a quick revision for their exams. The current concepts section of the book may inspire more exploration into this area.

It has been a pleasure to work with experts, both senior and junior, for this endeavor but we are particularly grateful to the publisher IntechOpen who have shown commitment and perseverance in completing this work. This new book deserves to be a success and we are sure it will be.

Amita Ray
Professor and Head of the Department of Obstetrics and Gynecology,
IQ City Medical College,
Durgapur, West Bengal, India

Section 1

Overview of Gestational Diabetes

Chapter 1

Introductory Chapter: Gestational Diabetes Mellitus

Amita Ray

1. The condition

Pregnancy, though a physiological condition, involves increased stress on a mother's biological processes. Advanced age, frequent pregnancies with shortened intervals, and several other risk factors may cause one of these processes to buckle under the stress giving rise to a disease state [1].

Gestational diabetes is a typical example which occurs as a temporary condition during pregnancy and is characterized by hyperglycemia and its varied manifestations. The word "gestational" implies exaggerated physiological response in pregnancy. Pregnancy is a state of insulin resistance, which has been designed by nature with the aim to supply the fetus with adequate nutrition at all times, irrespective of the mother's feeding cycles or habits. When this resistance, which is a physiological response to pregnancy, becomes aggravated and overcomes the pancreas capacity to secrete extra insulin, the result is a constant state of hyperglycemia. Risk factors and risk markers for GDM are age (the older a woman the higher her risk of GDM), overweight or obesity, excessive weight gain during pregnancy, a family history of diabetes, and GDM during a previous pregnancy [2].

Human placental lactogen and prolactin, the levels of which steadily increase during pregnancy, also contribute to the phenomena of increased insulin resistance by preventing the intake of insulin into peripheral tissue. A lesser explored hormone adiponectin exerts a protective effect by inhibiting hepatic glucose production. In GDM pregnancies, there is a significant decrease in placental adiponectin from an early stage of pregnancy, which now appears to be another independent risk factor for GDM. Adiponectin levels are also affected by pro-inflammatory cytokines, thus indicating a relationship between inflammation and carbohydrate metabolism or even a gross metabolic dysregulation [2].

2. The magnitude of the problem

According to the International Diabetes Federation (2017), 21.3 million or 16.2% of live births had some form of hyperglycemia in pregnancy, and a majority of these (85.1%) were due to gestational diabetes and one out of seven births is affected by gestational diabetes. The WHO Global Report on diabetes (2016) also gives similar figures: 75–90% of cases of hyperglycemia in pregnancy are due to gestational diabetes and 10–25% of pregnancies are affected by gestational diabetes. To complicate matters, a maximum number of these cases are from the low- and middle-income countries emphasizing the fact that diabetes per se as well as gestational diabetes are not the diseases of the affluent society who have access to quality health care [3]. A large number of these cases are from those sections of the population who do have access to basic antenatal care, where missing gestational diabetes is common and associated with grim outcomes for the mother and baby.

3. Maternal and fetal complications

Undetected, unmonitored, and uncontrolled gestational diabetes leads to severe maternal and fetal morbidity and mortality. GDM has a spectrum of both short- and long-term complications for both the mother and the fetus [4].

Among the short-term complications, are those that happen in the index pregnancy, hypertension is often associated with type 2 diabetes and so is true for GDM. Women who have GDM often develop hypertension during pregnancy and when compared to women who are euglycemic during pregnancy the difference is significant. Pregnancy-induced hypertension leads to several other problems in terms of preeclampsia and even eclampsia.

Several reasons for short-term morbidity in the mother are related to the increased size of the fetus. Nonprogress of labor and cephalopelvic disproportion due to a large-sized baby may lead to instrumental deliveries, perineal injuries, and C-sections.

For the fetus, the hallmark complication of GDM is macrosomia and the problems resulting from it. These could be sudden fetal demise, shoulder dystocia, obstructed labor, hydramnios, malpresentations, and cord prolapse. Macrosomia also leads to earlier onset of labor, giving rise to a preterm baby with all the associated risks of prematurity. The chief among these is the respiratory distress syndrome (RDS) due to lack of surfactant: this is a combined effect of prematurity as well as the fact that hyperglycemia per se also delays lung maturity.

The baby of a GDM mother has more chances of admission to intensive care due to RDS and also because it is more prone to metabolic derangements which are typical of this condition. Hypoglycemia, hyperbilirubinemia, and hypomagnesemia are significantly more in babies of GDM mothers.

When considering long-term complications of GDM recurrence of GDM in subsequent pregnancies and the development of type 2 diabetes in later life are the ones of major concern. A GDM mother has about 30–60% chance of recurrence in subsequent pregnancies. A systematic review of 28 studies covering the same number of years showed that a GDM mother has a cumulative incidence ranging from 2.6 to 70% of type 2 diabetes. Recurrence of GDM in subsequent pregnancies and the development of type 2 diabetes in later life are linked to risk factors like obesity, interval between pregnancies, and the amount of insulin needed during the index pregnancy.

Long-term complications in the neonate of a GDM mother are obesity and type 2 diabetes in adult life. The girl child also runs the risk of GDM in her pregnancy.

4. The controversies

Screening and diagnosis of gestational diabetes is varied and till date a single universal guideline has been elusive. This is compounded by the fact that both gestational diabetes and type 2 diabetes are very dependent on ethnicity. This often leads to the question as to whether a single mathematical figure would actually reflect hyperglycemia and its complications in different ethnic groups.

International and national bodies advise various ways to screen gestational diabetes. Large numbers of such guidelines confuse the primary health provider and the practicing obstetrician. In this era of evidence-based medicine, there is need for a single robust, evidence, practical guideline, the use of which would ensure the early detection and adequate management of gestational diabetes at the earliest in different countries and ethnic groups.

5. Recent advances

Although screening for GDM remains the mainstay for early detection, biomarkers for predicting, and monitoring the condition have also been identified. These biomarkers are altered as a result of the underlying pathology of GDM and thus help in predicting the condition before it actually becomes manifest clinically. These biomarkers may be related to insulin resistance, chronic inflammation, and altered placental function all of which are related to the patho-physiology of GDM. Micro-RNAs, one such group of biomarkers are a class of RNAs which are not involved in coding but can modulate gene expression. Thus, particular levels of circulating micro-RNAs can be used as biomarkers to predict GDM.

Efforts are also being made to combine several biomarkers to form a risk score for prediction of GDM. Combining clinical risk factors and biomarkers to predict the condition are also in the process.

6. The way ahead

Gestational diabetes mellitus has a well-documented link with maternal age, family history, diet, obesity, and lack of exercise. Both ethnicity and deprivation are major contributors to an increased risk of GDM. Research has confirmed that a better diet, increased physical activity, an appropriate pre-pregnancy Body Mass Index could reduce the development of gestational diabetes mellitus. The challenge now is to find ways of delivering these benefits in real life rather than in purely research settings. Keeping these things in mind, the first aim should be primary prevention. It plays the most significant role in creating awareness as regards gestational diabetes among public. Awareness should particularly target the groups which are at high risk for developing diabetes. Primary steps in preventing gestational diabetes can delay or halt further developments which in turn reduce both the need for gestational diabetes care and other required treatments. Prevention of gestational diabetes and diabetes per se should be considered a public health priority. The biggest task faced by the medical fraternity is lack of awareness across all segments of society about this epidemic.

A uniform consensus on how to screen for and diagnose gestational diabetes is another focus area for national and international bodies. As both ethnicity and deprivation are major contributors to this disease condition, the guidelines framed should make allowance for both [5, 6].

Another area that needs looking into is the identification of markers which could predict the condition with reasonable accuracy. It is also essential that such markers be cost-effective as both diabetes and gestational diabetes can no longer be considered as the disease of the elite society.

Author details

Amita Ray
Department of Obstetrics and Gynecology, IQ City Medical College, Durgapur, West Bengal, India

*Address all correspondence to: amitarays@gmail.com

References

[1] Kampmann U, Madsen LR, Skajaa GO, Iversen DS, Moeller N, Ovesen P. Gestational diabetes: A clinical update. World Journal of Diabetes. 2015;**6**(8):1065-1072

[2] Catalano PM, Hoegh M, Minium J, Huston-Presley L, Bernard S, Kalhan S, et al. Adiponectin in human pregnancy: Implications for regulation of glucose and lipid metabolism. Diabetologia. 2006;**49**(7):1677-1685

[3] Ferrara A. Increasing prevalence of gestational diabetes mellitus: A public health perspective. Diabetes Care. 2007;**30**(Suppl 2):S141-S146

[4] Yogev Y, Metzger BE. Hod MEstablishing diagnosis of gestational diabetes mellitus: Impact of the hyperglycemia and adverse pregnancy outcome study. Seminars in Fetal and Neonatal Medicine. 2009;**14**(2):94-100

[5] Jensen DM, Korsholm L, Ovesen P, Beck-Nielsen H, Mølsted-Pedersen L, Damm P. Adverse pregnancy outcome in women with mild glucose intolerance: Is there a clinically meaningful threshold value for glucose? Acta Obstetricia et Gynecologica Scandinavica. 2008;**87**: 59-62

[6] Metzger BE, Gabbe SG, Persson B, Buchanan TA, Catalano PA, Damm P, et al. International Association of Diabetes and Pregnancy Study Groups recommendations on the diagnosis and classification of hyperglycemia in pregnancy. Diabetes Care. 2010;**33**:676

Chapter 2

A Clinical Insight into Gestational Diabetes

HH Siddiqui, Tarique Mahmood, Mohd. Haris Siddiqui, Paramdeep Bagga, Farogh Ahsan and Arshiya Shamim

Abstract

Pregnancy is a diabetogenic state manifested by insulin resistance and hyperglycaemia. The age group at risk of getting gestational diabetes is between 20 and 39 years in 96.8% of cases. Gestational diabetes is the development of symptoms and signs of diabetes mellitus during pregnancy and the glucose level reverting to normal during puerperium. Depending on the type of population and the diagnostic criteria used, gestational diabetes is said to complicate 1–16% of all pregnancies. Many researchers in American, European and Asian surveys have reported 3–6% of prevalence. Compared with white European women, the prevalence rate for GD is increased approximately elevenfold in women from the Indian subcontinent, eightfold in South East Asia, sixfold and threefold in Arab and black Afro-Caribbean women, respectively. Such figures draw a potent clinical interest towards gestational diabetes (GD), and this chapter attempts to highlight some major aspects of GD in respect to both the mother and the foetus or the newborn specially emphasizing on its management as per the World Health Organization (WHO) and International Federation of Gynaecology and Obstetrics (FIGO).

Keywords: antenatal care, hyperinsulinaemia, impaired glucose tolerance, International Federation of gynaecology and obstetrics, medical nutrition therapy

1. Introduction

Gestational diabetes (GD) is characterised with impaired glucose tolerance (IGT) whose first recognition or onset is during pregnancy. International statistics claim that out of 10 pregnancies, at least 1 is associated with diabetes, most of which are GD. Lack 0f diagnosis or treatment of GD can lead to significant maternal and foetal complications. Moreover, women with GD and their offsprings are comparatively at higher risk of developing type 2 diabetes later [1–10].

The incidence of GD is expected to increase at an expedited rate in the near future, amounting to one in every five pregnant women suffering from GD. According to a field study conducted in one of the Indian states under the 'Diabetes in Pregnancy'—Awareness and Prevention project, in most of the pregnant women screened in urban, semiurban and rural areas, respectively, the prevalence of GD was reported to be 17.8% in the urban, 13.8% in the semiurban and 9.9% in the rural areas [11–16].

GD may result in development of many pregnancy-associated disorders like polyhydramnios, pre-eclampsia, prolonged labour, obstructed labour, caesarean section, uterine atony, postpartum haemorrhage, infection and progression of retinopathy which are the leading global causes of maternal morbidity and mortality.

Moreover, GD could also pose foetal risks including spontaneous abortion, intrauterine death, stillbirth, congenital malformation, birth injuries, neonatal hypoglycaemia and infant respiratory distress syndrome.

Long-term clinical effects of GD are important contributors to the burden of non-communicable diseases in many countries [17, 18].

2. Aetiology and pathophysiology of GD

During normal pregnancy, resistance to insulin action increases. In most pregnancies, the pancreas is able to meet the increased insulin demands, and normal blood glucose level is maintained. On the contrary, women who develop GD have impaired beta-cell response resulting in insufficient insulin secretion to meet the increased insulin demands. The following factors tend to enhance the chances of developing GD:

- Age: Due to age-related decreased pancreatic beta-cell reserve.
- Obesity: Leads to increased insulin resistance, which is further compounded by pregnancy.
- Smoking: Increases insulin resistance and decreases insulin secretion.
- Polycystic ovarian syndrome: Associated with insulin resistance and obesity.
- Nonwhite ancestry.
- Family history of type 2 diabetes.
- Intake of diet with low-fibre and high-glycaemic index.
- Weight gain.
- Lack of physical activity: Exercise increases insulin sensitivity.
- Prior GD: GD recurs in as many as 80% of subsequent pregnancies.

Products of the placenta, including tumour necrosis factor-alpha (TNF-α) and human chorionic somatomammotropin, are considered to play pathological roles in inducing maternal insulin resistance. Insulin resistance is observed at peak levels in the third trimester of pregnancy. Women who develop GD have pathologically impaired beta-cell function that leaves them with inability of adapting to pregnancy. In GD, as in type 2 diabetes, the deficit in beta-cell function is usually multifactorial and polygenetic. However, unmasked by the increased insulin needs of pregnancy, autoimmune diabetes and maturity-onset diabetes of youth (MODY) may occasionally be first recognised as GD. Hyperglycaemia in late pregnancy is associated with macrosomia and neonatal hypoglycaemia, hyperbilirubinemia and hypocalcaemia, as well as adverse maternal outcomes, including gestational hypertension, pre-eclampsia and caesarean delivery [19–35].

3. Strategical diagnosis of GD

Profound international evidences and standard protocols suggest definite guidelines for screening pregnant women for GD.

The American and Canadian guidelines recommend universal screening by two-step approach. This includes a screening with 50-g 1-hour blood glucose test (>140 mg/dL taken as screen positive). Women who screen positive are subjected to 100-g oral glucose tolerance test (OGTT), and those with 2 or more abnormal values of blood glucose are diagnosed with gestational diabetes.

Similarly, the National Institute for Health and Care Excellence (NICE), UK, and Australian guidelines recommend a slightly different risk-based screening. It recommends a 75-g 2-hour OGTT. Women with fasting blood glucose ≥126 mg/dL and postprandial (PP) blood glucose ≥140 mg/dL are diagnosed with GD [36, 37].

The WHO and International Federation of Gynaecology and Obstetrics (FIGO) endorse universal screening for GD at 24–28 weeks of gestation using the 75-g 2-hour blood sugar (fasting ≥126 mg/dL and PP ≥140 mg/dL).

Almost all guidelines agree to the management of GD using medical nutrition therapy (MNT) which is a standard diet plan for GD-diagnosed mothers and insulin therapy if required. Recently, global evidences have also concluded that the traditional biguanide—metformin—is safe and effective for GD management after 20 weeks of gestation if blood glucose level is not controlled alone by MNT [38–42].

GD pregnant women should be managed by medical nutrition therapy (MNT) and metformin or insulin therapy as required. In the postpartum period, OGTT must be repeated at 6 weeks post delivery; if blood glucose is <140 mg/dL, then women should be referred for postprandial blood glucose (PPBS) testing annually [43, 44].

3.1 Testing and management of GD

Ideally, all pregnant women should be screened for gestational diabetes, especially those who have one or more risk factors discussed above.

Trained human resources are required to manage the cases after diagnosis. Testing for GD is recommended twice during ante natal care (ANC).

The first testing should be done during the first antenatal contact as early as possible in pregnancy. If the first test result is negative, the test must be repeated between the second and third trimester of pregnancy. It is important to conduct a second test as most pregnant women develop blood glucose intolerance during this period (24–28 weeks). Mostly, one third of all GD-positive women are diagnosed during the first trimester. Hence, the test is repeated after the second trimester.

There should be at least a gap of 4 weeks between the two tests. The test should be conducted for all pregnant women even if she comes late in pregnancy for ANC. However, if the woman is over 28 weeks of pregnancy, only one test should be conducted if it is her first visit for ANC [45–51].

3.2 Methodology for diagnosis

The following stepwise protocol complies with the WHO guidelines for screening of pregnant women:

- The test is conducted with intake of 75 g of oral glucose dissolved in approximately 300 mL of water, irrespective of whether the pregnant woman comes in fasting or non-fasting state, followed by measuring the blood glucose level by a plasma-standardised glucometer after 2 hours of ingestion (postprandial blood glucose).

- If within 30 minutes of oral glucose intake the mother vomits, the test has to be repeated the next day. If vomiting occurs after 30 minutes, the test continues.

- The threshold blood glucose level of ≥140 mg/dL is considered as limit for diagnosis of GD [52–61].

4. Internationally acceptable guidelines for management of GD

4.1 Guiding principles

All pregnant women who screen positive for GD in the first test are subjected to medical nutrition therapy (MNT) and physical exercise for 2 weeks. The woman is advised to walk or exercise for at least 30 minutes a day.

After 2 weeks on MNT and physical exercise, a 2-hour PPBS (post meal) should be done. All standardised protocols for management of GD suggest initial management with MNT and physical exercise strictly. If diabetes is not controlled with MNT (lifestyle changes) alone, metformin or insulin therapy is recommended.

If 2-hour PPBS is <120 mg/dL, the test is to be repeated as per high-risk pregnancy protocol, i.e. to undertake eight tests (four regular tests and four additional). It is recommended to conduct at least one test every month during the second and third trimester. More follow-up tests can be done as recommended by the gynaecologist. If 2-hour PPBS is ≥120 mg/dL, medical management (metformin or insulin therapy) has to be started as per guidelines (**Figure 1**) [62–66].

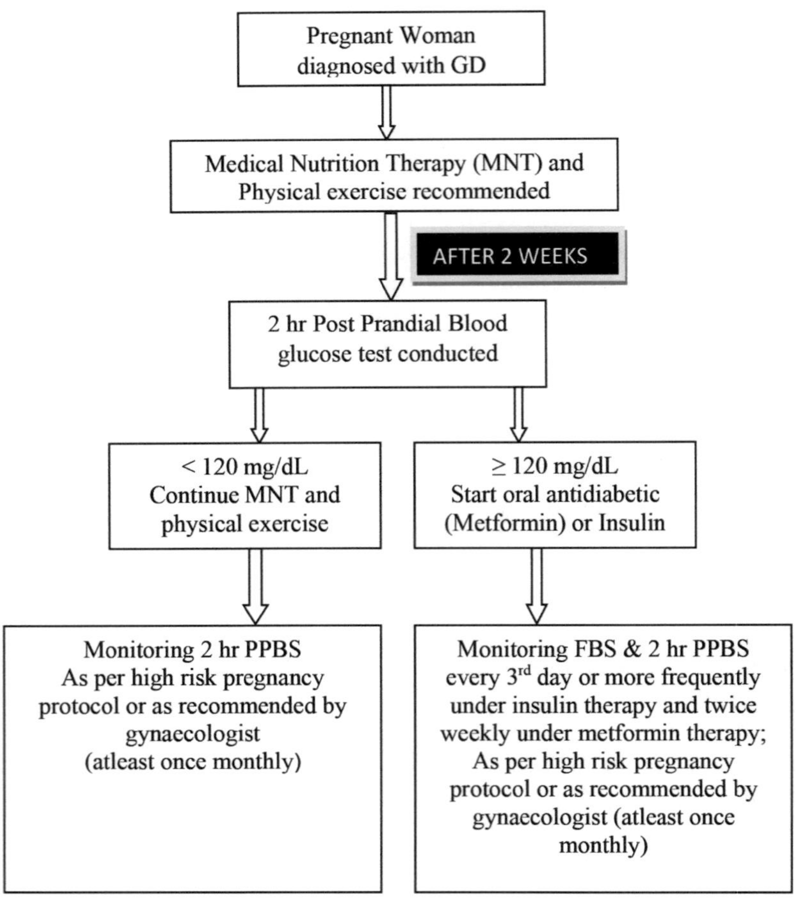

Figure 1.
Standard health management protocol for pregnant women with GD.

4.2 Medical nutrition therapy (MNT)

4.2.1 Healthy eating during pregnancy

All pregnant women with GD should get medical nutrition therapy (MNT) as soon as diagnosis is made. MNT for GD primarily involves a carbohydrate-controlled balanced meal plan which promotes:

- Optimal nutrition for maternal and foetal health
- Adequate energy for appropriate gestational weight gain
- Achievement and maintenance of normoglycaemia [67, 68]

4.3 The significance of the individualised nutrition plan assessment in GD

Assessment of diet or nutrition plan in GD is an important criterion for diagnosis and subsequent follow-up on mother's and foetus' development. The nutrition plan must be individualised from patient to patient so that accurate appraisal of the woman's nutritional status could be assessed. This assessment includes defining her body mass index (BMI) or percentage of desirable weight during pre-pregnancy to the optimal weight gain during the entire tenure of pregnancy [24, 69].

4.4 Monitoring calorie intake in GD

The energy demand of the body during pregnancy increases many times than that in a nonpregnant state. Individualization of nutritional requirement proves to be very helpful in determining the energy requirement and making amendments in the diet plan based on weight change patterns.

Normally calorie monitoring is not a point of concern in the first trimester unless a woman is underweight. It becomes more significant during the second and third trimester to monitor the energy requirements. Calorie intake should suffice the appropriate weight gain during gestation.

Ideally, for an average woman, weight gain of 10–12 kg is considered normal during pregnancy; an additional 350 kcal/day intake to the adult requirement is recommended during the second and third trimester.

Severe caloric restriction is strictly prohibited as it may cause ketonaemia and ketonuria in the mother as well as impair physical and mental growth in the offspring (**Tables 1** and **2**) [70–72].

Energy requirement can be calculated as follows:

$$\text{Energy requirement (kcal/day)} = \text{BMR} \times \text{PAL} \tag{1}$$

*BMR = basal metabolic rate; *PAL = physical activity level.

where the basal metabolic rate (BMR) for an adult female in the age group of 18–30 years is calculated as 14 × BW (kg) + 471 and similarly BMR for adult females of age group 30–60 years as 8.3 × BW (kg) + 788 (**BW = body weight*).

4.4.1 Daily intake of carbohydrates

Carbohydrates are essential for both the mother and the baby. They are the ultimate source of glucose in the blood. Hence, the nature, quantity and frequency of carbohydrate intake influence greatly the blood glucose level.

S. no.	Nature of lifestyle	Energy requirement during pregnancy	Total energy requirement (kcal/day)
1.	Sedentary	1900 + 350	2250
2.	Moderately active	2230 + 350	2580
3.	Highly active	2850 + 350	3200

Table 1.
Energy requirement in relation to nature of lifestyle.

S. no.	Body mass index	Calorie requirement
1.	<18.5 (underweight)	Calorie requirement as per activity + 500 kcal/day
2.	18.5–22.9 (normal)	Calorie requirement as per activity
3.	23–24.9 (overweight)	Calorie requirement as per activity
4.	>25 (obese)	Calorie requirement as per activity—500 kcal/day

Table 2.
Calorie requirement according to body mass index (BMI).

The carbohydrates must be evenly distributed through the daily food chart foods in order to avoid high blood glucose level. It is better to spread carbohydrate foods over three small meals and two to three snacks each day than taking three large meals [8, 73–78].

Complex carbohydrates (like whole-grain cereals like oats, vegetables and fruits) should be preferred over simple carbohydrates like food with lots of added sugar or honey. Also keeping a record of the number of carbohydrate serves that a mother eats during the day helps her to eat the right amount of carbohydrates [79].

4.4.2 Daily intake of fats

Overall fat intake by a pregnant woman should be planned in a manner that saturated fat such as butter, coconut oil, palm oil, red meat, organ meat and full cream milk amounts to less than 10% of total calories. The dietary cholesterol must be less than 300 mg/dL. In obese and overweight patients, a lower-fat diet overall can help slow the rate of weight gain [80].

4.4.3 Daily intake of proteins

Proteins are a very important dietary element for the growth and health of the foetus.

At least three servings of protein foods are recommended every day to meet the increased demand. Milk and milk products, egg, fish, chicken, pulses, nuts, etc. are all rich sources of protein that a mother can take during her pregnancy [80].

5. Pharmacotherapy of GD with metformin and insulin

The widely accepted treatment protocol for gestational diabetes advocates metformin or insulin therapy for clinical management of pregnant women diagnosed with GD that is not well controlled with MNT alone. Insulin is the first drug of choice for GD mothers.

The advantage of insulin therapy over metformin is that it can be started any time during pregnancy for GD management. If the gestation is less than 20 weeks, and medical nutrition therapy (MNT) is not effective in controlling blood glucose levels, insulin should be started, but metformin can be considered only after 20 weeks of gestation for clinical management of GD.

Metformin therapy can be started at 20 weeks of pregnancy, if MNT has not been able to control blood glucose alone. In the cases where the woman's blood glucose is not controlled even with the maximum dose of metformin and MNT, the therapy must be switched to insulin therapy. The dose of metformin is 500 mg BID orally up to a maximum dose up to 2 g/day.

The incidence of hypoglycaemia and weight gain with metformin is less than insulin. If insulin is required in high doses, metformin may be added to the treatment. Any pregnant women on insulin therapy should be instructed to keep sugar/glucose powder handy at home to treat hypoglycaemia if it occurs [81–84].

5.1 Common side effects with metformin

- Diarrhoea
- Nausea
- Stomach pain
- Heartburn
- Lactic acidosis
- Low blood glucose

5.2 Types of insulins

Unlike the nonpregnant patients with diabetes who have a plethora of choices to achieve glucose control, the pregnant cases with GD offer a big challenge to the clinicians when it comes to the choice of drugs for its management. In the recent years, we have come across a variety in new insulins, novel delivery systems and additional concentrations of existing insulins. With an alarming increase in the gestational diabetic population, the demands of the newer insulins will be ever increasing; hence, understanding these insulins becomes crucial. Additional pharmacokinetic and pharmacodynamic studies of these insulins in pregnancy are also required [85].

5.2.1 Short-acting insulin and rapid-acting insulin analogues

5.2.1.1 Regular (U-100) insulin

It is identical to human insulin and is synthesised in *Escherichia coli* bacteria. It is used before meal to compensate for heavy carbohydrates. The onset of action is around 30 minutes but can range from 10 to 75 minutes. The peak action is achieved at 3 hours (range 20 minutes to 7 hours), and the overall duration of action is ~8 hours. U-100 vials can stay at room temperature for 31 days [86].

5.2.1.2 Regular (U-500) insulin

It is identical to human insulin but more concentrated than the U-100 formulation; its pharmacokinetic profile differs from U-100 as well. The onset is ~30 minutes, but the duration of action can last up to 24 hours. Severe hypoglycaemia may occur 24 hours after the initial dose, although there are clinical reports suggesting that in pregnancy, severe hypoglycaemia is rare with U-500 insulin. Two to three injections daily are required, and a U-500 vial is good for 40 days at room temperature while in use [87–89].

5.2.1.3 Insulin aspartate

It is produced in a type of yeast, *Saccharomyces cerevisiae*, and is homologous to human insulin. It should be taken 5–10 minutes prior to meals. It can be administered as injections or in an insulin pump. The time of peak concentration ranges between 40 and 50 minutes, and the duration of action is 3–5 hours. It is also available in the forms of pens, penfills and vials that retain their pharmacological potency for at least 28 days at room temperature while in use. The risk of developing hypoglycaemia with insulin aspartate is less than regular insulin, although patients allergic to yeast must avoid it as this could potentially cause a site reaction [90].

5.2.1.4 Insulin lispro (U-100 and U-200)

It is an analogue produced in *Escherichia coli*. Its onset of action is 10–15 minutes, peak action is attained in 30–90 minutes and the duration of action is 3–4 hours. Intraperitoneal injections are preferred for the maximum absorption and shortest duration of action. It can be used in the form of insulin pumps or as multiple daily injections. The U-100 and U-200 formulations are bioequivalent, having the same pharmacokinetics. Insulin lispro U-200 is only available in pens to avoid administration errors. Pens, penfills and vials can be stored for 28 days at room temperature while in use [91].

5.2.2 Intermediate insulin and long-acting insulin analogues

5.2.2.1 Insulin isophane (NPH)

It is a U-100, intermediate-acting insulin. It is produced in *Escherichia coli* and is identical to human insulin available as a suspension. The onset of action is 1–2 hours, with an average peak action of 4 hours (range, 4–8 hours). Duration of action lasts for 10–20 hours. Vials remain usable for 31 days at room temperature, whereas pens can be used for 14 days [92].

5.2.2.2 Insulin detemir (U-100)

This is a long-acting analogue of insulin produced in *S. cerevisiae*. One of the setbacks with this formulation is that it can potentially cause a reaction in patients who are allergic to yeast. Detemir lacks a defined peak of action, but the pharmacological action lasts for up to 20 hours. The time to onset of action ranges between 1 and 2 hours. The pen and vial can be used up to 42 days at room temperature while in use. The chances of developing hypoglycaemia with detemir are less than NPH in pregnant women [93].

5.2.2.3 Insulin glargine (U-100)

It is a long-acting analogue produced in *Escherichia coli*. It differs from other contemporaries in terms of its distribution in plasma; the acidic solution is neutralised in subcutaneous tissue to form microprecipitates. These microprecipitates slowly release glargine over a duration of 24 hours, resulting in no well-defined peak. Its onset of action is 1–2 hours. Vials and pens are reusable for 28 days at room temperature.

5.2.2.4 Insulin degludec U-100 and U-200

They are long-acting analogues approved by the US Food and Drug Administration (FDA) in September 2015. The U-100 and the U-200 are considered bioequivalent. Insulin degludec is extracted by means of recombinant DNA technology implemented in *S. cerevisiae*, to avoid potential reaction to the yeast, if allergic. Insulin degludec's slow absorption into blood and prolonged action are attributed to the formation of soluble multi-hexamers. Its onset of action is ~1 hour and takes 8 days to reach steady state, and, once achieved, its duration of action lasts for 42 hours. It is usually administered once daily at any time of the day due to its long duration of action. Noncompliant patients may inject their dose at intervals of 8–40 hours without significant decreases in glycosylated haemoglobin (HbA1C) compared to taking it at the same time every day. U-100 degludec and U-200 degludec are only dispensed in pens to decrease administration errors. Pens are good for up to 56 days at room temperature while in use [93].

5.3 Novel drug delivery system for insulin

Insulin in the form of inhalational powder is a newer form of insulin introduced in recent years. Human insulin inhalation powder was approved by the FDA in 2014. Inhaled human insulin is produced in *Escherichia coli* and is adsorbed onto fumaryl diketopiperazine and polysorbate 80 carrier particles. Inhalation powder is equivalent unit for unit to insulin lispro. Its onset is 12–15 minutes, and it takes ~57 minutes to reach peak levels in plasma. The duration of action is ~2 hours. Inhaled human insulin is contraindicated in patients with chronic pulmonary obstructive disease as it may precipitate chronic bronchospasm. Sealed blister cards at room temperature must be discarded after 10 days. If kept in the refrigerator, they are good for use up to 1 month (**Figure 2**) [94, 95].

5.4 Glyburides-new hypoglycaemic drugs

A new advent in the field of glucose-lowering agents is glyburides. It is an oral hypoglycaemic class of drugs used for the management of type-II diabetes mellitus. Pharmacologically it belongs to sulphonylurea class of insulin secretagogues. These agents stimulate β cells of the pancreas to release insulin. The members of this class have different binding sites on their target pancreatic β-cell receptor. Their dose, rate of absorption, duration of action and route of elimination also differ from the conventional hypoglycaemic agents. Apart from lowering the blood glucose level directly, glyburide also increases peripheral glucose utilisation, decreases hepatic gluconeogenesis and may increase the number and sensitivity of insulin receptors. Glyburides proved to be advantageous over insulin because weight gain associated with it is less than in the case of insulin. However, one of its fallacies is that it may cause hypoglycaemia and require consistent food intake to decrease this risk. The risk of hypoglycaemia is increased in elderly, debilitated and malnourished individuals. Glyburide has been shown to decrease fasting plasma glucose, postprandial blood glucose and glycosylated haemoglobin (HbA1c) levels. It is metabolised in the liver. Its metabolites are excreted in urine and faeces in approximately equal proportions [96].

5.4.1 Indication

It is prescribed to be taken at meal time to lower the blood glucose level in patients with non-insulin-dependent diabetes mellitus where hyperglycaemia cannot be controlled by diet alone.

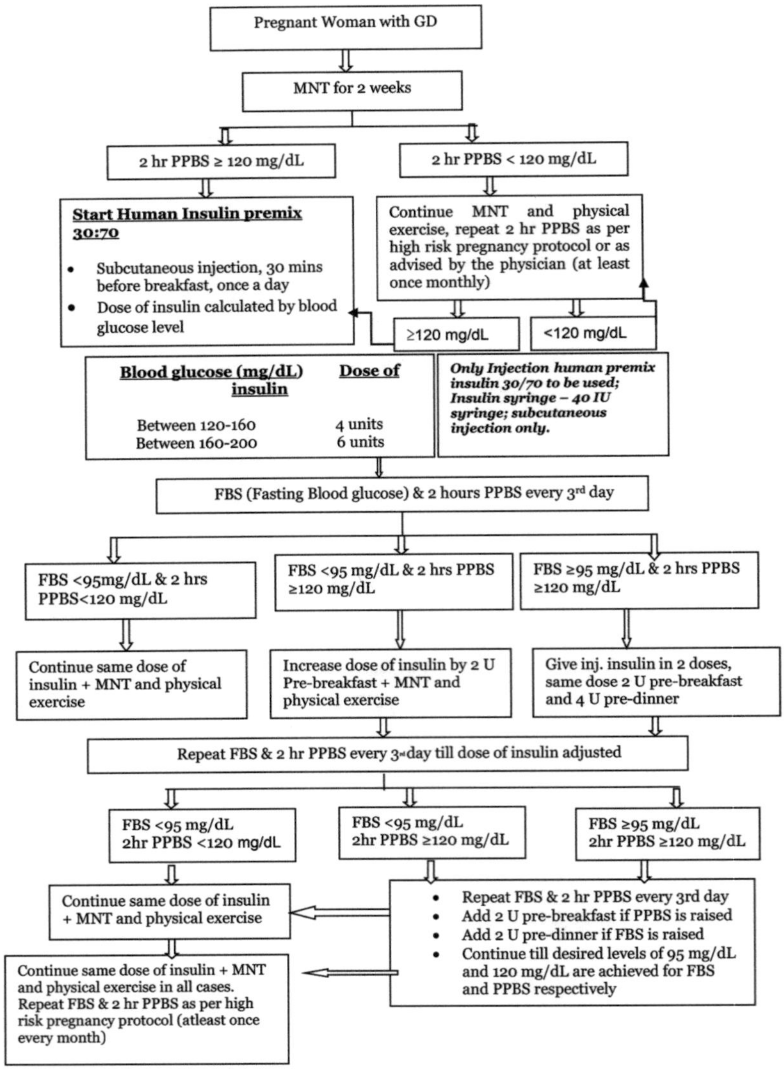

Figure 2.
Insulin therapy for GD.*

5.4.2 Half-life (t 1/2) and duration of action

The half-life of unchanged drug lies between 1 and 2 hours and its metabolites have an extended half-life of 10 hours. Duration of action is 12–24 hours.

5.4.3 Side effects

Nausea, heartburn, stomach fullness and weight gain may occur.

5.4.4 Precautions

- Contraindicated in hypersensitive patients.
- Given the high risk of hypoglycaemia associated with it. Patients must be counselled to avoid driving, the use of machinery or any activity that requires alertness or clear vision as low blood glucose levels may cause drowsiness, fatigue and blurred vision.

- Alcohol intake must be avoided under its medication as it aggravates hypoglycaemia and may cause disulfiram-like reaction.
- Older adults may be more sensitive to the side effects of this drug, especially low blood sugar.
- During pregnancy, this medication should be used only when clearly needed. Pregnancy may cause or worsen diabetes.

Hypoglycaemia	Considerations
Criteria	• *Mild hypoglycaemia:* Blood glucose level is <4.0 mmol/L and may or may not be associated with symptoms of a low blood glucose level • *Severe hypoglycaemia:* Blood glucose level is very low, generally <3.0 mmol/L, and is associated with confusion and potential loss of consciousness. The woman requires third-party assistance to manage the episode
Causes	• Extensive physical activity • Insulin overdose • Lack or inadequate carbohydrate in meal • Alcohol consumption (decreases blood glucose)
Symptoms	• Hunger • Light headedness/headache • Sweating/shaking/weakness • Tingling around the lips • Irritability • Blurred vision • Severe hypoglycaemia (when unable to self-treat) can lead to confusion and loss of consciousness and requires urgent medical treatment
Treatment	• Consume one 15-g serve of fast-acting carbohydrates (one of the following) • 5–7 glucose candies • Glass of soft drink rich in calories • Three-heaped teaspoons of sugar or honey dissolved in water • If after 15 minutes symptoms persist or BGL is less than 4.0 mmol/L, repeat one serve of fast-acting carbohydrates • Do not overtreat with fast-acting carbohydrates as this may lead to rebound hyperglycaemia • When BGL is 4.0 mmol/L or above, eat longer-lasting carbohydrate • Eat a snack (e.g. sandwich or glass of milk) or usual meal if within 30 minutes • Avoid overtreatment of hypoglycaemia resulting in hyperglycaemia • Document BGL and time of hypoglycaemic episode
Lifestyle management	• Plan to eat regular meals with adequate carbohydrate serves • Be prepared and carry a food snack at all times (including while exercising) • Aim to take long- or intermediate-acting insulin at the same time each day • Identify causal factors of the hypoglycaemic episode and avoid/mitigate for the future • Carry blood glucose metre at all times so BGL can be checked if symptoms present

Table 3.
Aspects surrounding hypoglycaemia in women under oral hypoglycaemic drugs or insulin.

- If glyburide is used, it may be switched to insulin at least 2 weeks before the expected delivery date because of glyburide's risk of causing low blood sugar in your newborn.
- It is unknown if this medication passes into breast milk. However, similar drugs pass into breast milk [97].

5.5 Monitoring blood glucose levels in GD mothers

The blood glucose monitoring in gestational diabetic cases remains a bone of contention amongst clinicians worldwide. There have been various cohort studies propounding different procedures for blood glucose level monitoring. Some suggest the evaluation of HbA_{1C} levels as accurate parameter; others suggest ultrasonography and laboratory testing of postprandial blood glucose levels every 2 weeks. For women whose fasting blood glucose levels remain <105 md/dL are well managed alone with medical nutrition therapy, whereas for those whose blood glucose levels are >105 mg/dL require additional medical assistance including insulin therapy. The foetal abdominal circumference (AC) is also considered a pivotal parameter for monitoring the GD mothers. If the foetal AC is <70th percentile at 30 weeks, perinatal outcomes will be free from any complications with continued management on diet therapy and without glucose self-monitoring. The excess risk of macrosomia is attributed to women with a foetal AC >70th percentile at 30 weeks. Such pregnancies will benefit only from aggressive glucose lowering by insulin therapy. The fasting or preprandial glucose targets of 60–80 mg/dL have to be met in such cases to eliminate the excess risk of stillbirth [98–101].

5.6 Hypoglycaemia

Hypoglycaemia is uncommon in women with GD who are only on MNT; the risk of developing hypoglycaemia is however increased in women on pharmacotherapy, i.e. insulin or metformin. Hypoglycaemia incurs potent hazards to the health of the foetus. Hence, management of hypoglycaemia is also a crucial aspect in GD. If hypoglycaemia is asymptomatic, BGL results must be confirmed prior to starting the treatment (**Table 3**) [102].

6. Special obstetric care for pregnant women with GD

6.1 Antenatal care (ANC)

Antenatal care is defined as the procedure of regular check-ups that allow clinicians to treat and prevent potential health problems throughout the course of the pregnancy and to promote healthy lifestyles that benefit both the mother and child. In the case of pregnant women with GD, they must be closely monitored. GD women who are diagnosed before 20 weeks of pregnancy undergo foetal anatomical survey by means of ultrasonography within 18–20 weeks of pregnancy.

At 28–30 weeks of gestation, a foetal growth scan should be performed and repeated at 34–36 weeks of gestation. There should be at least 3-week gap between the two ultrasounds, and it should include foetal biometry and amniotic fluid estimation.

In GD women having uncontrolled blood glucose level or any other complication of pregnancy, the antenatal visits should be programmed at least once monthly as per the protocol for high-risk pregnancy.

Monitoring of abnormal foetal growth and amniotic fluid volume for growth restriction and polyhydramnios, respectively, at each ANC visit is clinically important. Pregnant women with GD should be diligently monitored for gestational hypertension, proteinuria and other obstetric complications.

Antenatal steroids in pregnant women with GD between 24 and 34 weeks of gestation requiring early delivery should be administered as per standardised guidelines. Most guidelines like FIGO suggest dexamethasone injection. More vigilant monitoring of blood glucose levels should be done for the next 72 hours following injection. In the case of raised blood glucose levels during this period, adjustment of insulin dose should be made as required [103–105].

6.2 Monitoring foetal health in pregnant women with GD

The rate of foetal morbidity in pregnant women with GD is more than the normal ones. This risk is further accelerated in pregnant women under drug management. Hence vigilant foetal surveillance is required that includes foetal heart rate monitoring by auscultation on each antenatal care visit [105, 106].

6.3 Management of parturition in the case of GD

Pregnant women with GD but well controlled of blood glucose (2-hour PPBS <120 mg/dL) levels may be delivered at their respective health facility just like any normal pregnant woman. However, pregnant women with GD on insulin therapy with uncontrolled blood glucose levels (2-hour PPBS ≥120 mg/dL) on MNT and physical exercise and metformin or insulin requirement >20 U/day should be referred at 34–36 weeks for delivery planning at Comprehensive Emergency Obstetric Care (CEmOC) centres under supervision of a gynaecologist [107].

6.4 Timing of delivery

Most GD pregnancies are associated with delayed lung maturity of the foetus; hence routine delivery prior to 39 weeks is not recommended. Such referred cases must get assured indoor admission or can be kept in a birth waiting home with round-the-clock availability of gynaecologist for monitoring.

Managing the delivery timing in GD mother is very crucial if pregnant women with GD and well-controlled blood glucose have not undergone parturition spontaneously; induction of labour should be scheduled at or after 39 weeks of pregnancy.

If pregnant women with GD present poor blood glucose levels, accompanied with risk factors like gestational hypertension, previous stillbirth and other complications, then the timing of delivery has to be individualised by the obstetrician accordingly.

Vaginal delivery is preferred, and lower segment caesarean section (LSCS) is done for obstetric indications only such as in the case of foetal macrosomia, a condition where the estimated foetal weight is >4 kg where vaginal delivery may cause shoulder dystocia in the newborn.

Regular blood glucose monitoring of the pregnant women with GD on metformin or insulin is required during labour. The morning dose of insulin/metformin is withheld on the day of induction of labour, and pregnant women are subjected to 2 hourly monitoring of blood glucose.

IV infusion with normal saline (NS) is to be started and regular insulin to be added according to blood glucose levels as per **Table 4** [105–108].

Blood glucose level	Amount of insulin to be added in 500 mL of NS	Rate of NS infusion
90–120 mg/dL	0	100 ml/hour (16 drops/min)
120–140 mg/dL	4 U	100 ml/hour (16 drops/min)
140–180 mg/dL	6 U	100 ml/hour (16 drops/min)
>180 mg/dL	8 U	100 ml/hour (16 drops/min)

Table 4.
Rate and amount of insulin-normal saline infusion in relation to blood glucose level.

6.4.1 Neonatal care for baby of a GD mother

Immediate and timely management of all neonates in a proper NICU facility emphasising on early breastfeeding is done on a priority basis to prevent hypoglycaemia. Under any emergency situations, the sick neonates must be immediately resuscitated as per standard guidelines.

Hypoglycaemia monitoring of the newborn is started within an hour of delivery and repeated every 4 hours (prior to next feed) until four stable glucose values are obtained.

The newborn with the normal birth weight and blood glucose level of <45 mg/dL is considered hypoglycaemic and requires immediate medical management. In the case of intrauterine growth restriction (IUGR), newborns' Blood Glucose level limit is <54 mg/dL [108].

6.4.2 Diagnosis of hypoglycaemia

The glucometers' testing method is not very reliable for diagnosis of hypoglycaemia as their precision decreases at lower blood glucose level. The most definite diagnosis of hypoglycaemia is by measurement of blood glucose using established laboratory methods such as glucose oxidase method by calorimeter. However, if laboratory facility is unavailable at the place of childbirth, then the treating physician can take a decision to send a blood glucose sample to the laboratory at the nearest location without delaying the next management step. However, under adverse circumstances, blood glucose values obtained by glucometers may be considered for all operational steps if it's the question of newborn's wellbeing.

6.4.3 Symptoms of hypoglycaemia

Symptoms of hypoglycaemia are difficult to observe as in most cases it is asymptomatic, variable and observed only in a smaller proportion of patients or newborns:

- Stupor or apathy
- Jitteriness or tremors
- Episodes of cyanosis
- Convulsions
- Intermittent apnoeic spells or tachypnoea
- Weak and high-pitched cry, limpness and lethargy

- Difficulty in feeding
- Eye rolling
- Episodes of sweating
- Any unexplained clinical feature in baby of diabetic mother

6.4.4 Management of hypoglycaemia in newborn

All cases of newborn with hypoglycaemia should be managed in the following manner:

6.4.4.1 Step 1

Whether there are any symptoms of hypoglycaemia or not, if a baby is born to a GD mother, its blood glucose level must be checked immediately between 1 and 2 hours after birth. If blood glucose values are <45 mg/dL, this should be considered as 'hypoglycaemia'. The primary management in such cases is that the newborn should be given breastfeed without any delay. Direct breastfeeding is the best management step for neonatal hypoglycaemia. If the infant is unable to suck, expressed breast milk from the mother should be given. If the mother is not in a position to give breastfeed or in the case of no breast milk secretion, the baby should be given any formula feed. If the lactation management centres (human milk banks) are available at the facility, then it can also be involved in feeding the baby.

After an hour of breastfeeding the newborn, blood glucose level must be monitored again. If it is found to be more than 45 mg/dL, 2 hourly feeding (breastfeeding if not available, formula feed can be given) should be ensured by explaining to the mother/relatives and supervised.

6.4.4.2 Step 2

If at any point of time the blood glucose level drops below 20 mg/dL, immediate intravenous bolus injection of 10% dextrose at 2 mL/kg body weight of baby should be given. This should be followed by intravenous infusion of 10% of dextrose at a rate of 100 mL/kg/day. Blood glucose should be checked 30 minutes after starting the infusion. If it is still less than 20 mg/dL, the infant should be referred to a higher centre where a paediatrician is available [109, 110].

6.4.5 Postdelivery follow-up of pregnant women with GD

Immediate postpartum care required for women with GD is a lot similar to that for women without GD, but these women are at high risk to develop type 2 diabetes mellitus in the future, although in 80% of cases, the glucose level usually returns to normal postdelivery.

Subsequently, ANC must be performed 75-g OGTT (fasting and 2-hour PP) at 6 weeks postpartum to evaluate glycaemic status of a woman. Cut-off for normal plasma and abnormal blood glucose levels in the fasting and 75-g OGTT values are [111–113]:

- Fasting blood glucose (≥126 mg/dL)
- 75-g OGTT (2-hour blood glucose)

- Normal (<140 mg/dL)
- IGT (140–199 mg/dL)
- Diabetes (≥200 mg/dL)

7. Conclusion

This chapter summarises all the clinical aspects surrounding gestational diabetes, ranging from its pathophysiology, aetiology right to its proper clinical management, for both the mother and the newborn, to a GD mother. Pregnancy affects both the maternal and foetal metabolisms, and even the nondiabetic woman exerts a diabetogenic effect. Amongst pregnant women, 2–17.8% develop GD. Metabolic changes in the normal pregnant women also have a degree of insulin resistance that shunts glucose preferentially to the foetus. To maintain blood glucose levels within a tight range, the normal pregnant woman must increase her insulin secretion up to fourfold. When the pancreas is not able to compensate for the increased insulin needs of pregnancy, GD occurs resulting in hyperglycaemia and hyperinsulinemia.

Acknowledgements

The authors are highly thankful to Prof. S.W. Akhtar, Hon'ble Chancellor Integral University, and Prof. Syed Misbahul Hasan, Dean of the Faculty of Pharmacy, Integral University, Lucknow, India, for providing an academically rich environment in the university's infrastructure to explore and study extensively into clinically relevant fields.

Conflict of interest

The authors declare that there are no 'conflicts of interest' in regard to this chapter's contents.

Notes/thanks/other declarations

None.

List of abbreviations

ANC	antenatal care
BMI	body mass index
BMR	basal metabolic rate
CEmOC	comprehensive emergency obstetric care
GD	gestational diabetes
IGT	impaired glucose tolerance
IUGR	intrauterine growth restriction
LSCS	lower segment caesarean section
MNT	medical nutrition therapy
NCD	non-communicable diseases
OGTT	oral glucose tolerance test
PPBS	postprandial blood sugar

Author details

HH Siddiqui[1], Tarique Mahmood[2†], Mohd. Haris Siddiqui[1], Paramdeep Bagga[2], Farogh Ahsan[2] and Arshiya Shamim[2*†]

1 Faculty of Pharmacy, Integral University, Lucknow, India

2 Department of Bioengineering, Integral University, Lucknow, India

*Address all correspondence to: arshiyas@iul.ac.in

† These authors have equally contributed in structuring the chapter.

References

[1] Colagiuri S, Sandbaek A, Carstensen B, Christensen J, Glumert C, Lauritzen T, et al. Comparability of venous and capillary glucose measurements in blood. Diabetic Medicine. 2003;**20**:953-956

[2] Farrar D, Duley L, Dowswell T, Lawlor DA. Different strategies for diagnosing gestational diabetes to improve maternal and infant health. Cochrane Database of Systematic Reviews. 2017(8)

[3] Harlting L, Dryden D, Guthrie A, Muise M, Vandermeer B, Aktary W, et al. Screening and Diagnosing Gestational Diabetes: Evidence Report/ Technology Assessment. Agency for Healthcare Research and Quality: U.S. Department of Health and Human Services. No. 210; 2012

[4] International Diabetes Federation. South-East Asia: IDF Diabetes Atlas. 2012. Available from: http://www.idf.org/diabetesatlas/5e/south-east-asia

[5] Jiwani A, Marseille E, Lohse N, Damm P, Hod M, Kahn J. Gestational diabetes: Results from a survey of country prevalence and practices. Journal of Maternal-Fetal and Neonatal Medicine. 2012;**25**(6):600-610

[6] Khan KS, Wojdlya D, Say L, Gulmezoglu AM, Van Look PF. WHO analysis of causes of maternal death: A systematic review. Lancet. 2006;**367**(9516):1066-1074

[7] Priya M, Anhan R, Pradeepa R, Jayashuri R, Deepa M, Bhansali A, et al. Comparison of capillary whole blood versus venous plasma glucose estimations in screening for diabetes mellitus in epidemiological studies in developing countries. Diabetes Technology & Therapeutics. 2011;**13**:586-591

[8] Seshiah V, Balaji V, Vitull G, Anil K. Gestational diabetes: The public health relevance and approach. Diabetes Research and Clinical Practice. 2012;**97**:350-358

[9] Seshiah V, Balaji V, Balaji MS, Paneerselvam A, Kapur A. Pregnancy and diabetes scenario around the world: India. International Journal of Gynecology & Obstetrics. 2009;**104**(Suppl. 1):S35-S38

[10] Seshiah V, Balaji V, Balaji M, Sanjeevi C, Green A. Gestational diabetes in India. The Journal of the Association of Physicians of India. 2004;**52**:707-711

[11] Kragelund NK, Damm P, Kapur A, Balaji V, Balaji MS, Seshiah V, et al. Risk factors for hyperglycaemia in pregnancy in Tamil Nadu, India. PLoS One. 2016;**11**(3):e0151311. DOI: 10.1371/journal.pone.0151311

[12] Crowther CA, Hiller JE, Moss JR, et al. Effects of treatment of gestational diabetes on pregnancy outcomes. The New England Journal of Medicine. 2005;**352**:2477-2486

[13] Langer O. Maternal glycemic criteria for insulin therapy in gestational diabetes. Diabetes Care. 1998;**21**(Suppl 2):B91

[14] Mangesi L, Hofmeyr GJ, Smith V, Smyth RM. Fetal movement counting for assessment of fetal wellbeing. Cochrane Database of Systematic Reviews. 2015(10)

[15] McFarland MB, Langer O, Conway DL, et al. Dietary therapy for gestational diabetes: How long is long enough? Obstetrics and Gynecology. 2005;**93**:978

[16] Moore TR, Catalano P. Chapter 46: Diabetes in pregnancy. In: Creasy RK, Resnik R, et al., editors. Maternal-Fetal Medicine: Principles and Practice. 6th ed. ELsevier Inc. 2009. pp. 953-993

[17] World Health Organisation (WHO). Diet, Nutrition and the Prevention of Chronic Diseases. Technical Report Series 916; 2003

[18] Pridjian G. Pregestational Diabetes in Obs. & Gynae Clinics of North America (Update on Medical Disorders in Pregnancy); June 2010, Vol. 37. No. 2. BS-143-158. Saunders & Elsevier Inc; 2010

[19] Pridjian G, Benjamine TD. Gestational Diabetes in Obs & Gynae Clinics of North America (Update on Medical Disorders in Pregnancy); June 2010, Vol. 37. No. 2. BS-257-267. Saunders & Elsevier Inc; 2010

[20] Nainggolon L. ACOG new practice bulletin on gestational diabetes. Obstetrics Gynaecology. 2013;**122**:BS 406-416

[21] Diagnostic Criteria & Classification of Hyperglycemia First Detected in Pregnancy. World Health Organization; 2013

[22] Berger H, Crane J, Faisal D, et al. Screening for gestational diabetes. In: SOGC Clinical Practice Guidelines No. 12. 2002

[23] Nankervis A, Mc Intyre HD, Moses R, et al. ADIPS Consensus Guidelines for the Testing & Diagnosis of Gestational Diabetes in Austria. 2013

[24] HAPO Collaboration Research Group. Hyperglycemia & adverse pregnancy outcomes. The New England Journal of Medicine. 2008;**358**:1991-2002

[25] IADPSG Consensus Panel. International association of diabetes & pregnancy study groups recommendations on the diagnosis & classification of hyperglycemia in pregnancy. Diabetes Care. 2010;**33**:676-682

[26] American Diabetes Association. Standard of medical care in diabetes. Diabetes Care. 2011;**34**(suppl 1):S11-S61

[27] Diabetes in Pregnancy-NICE Clinical Guidelines Issued by National Institute for Health & Clinical Excellence; 2008

[28] Rowan JA, Hague WM, Gao W, Battin MR, Moore MP. Metformin versus insulin for the treatment of gestational diabetes. The New England Journal of Medicine. 2008;**358**:2003-2015

[29] Gui J, Liu Q, Feng L. Metformin vs insulin in the management of gestational diabetes: A meta-analysis. PLoS One. 2013;**8**:e64585

[30] Seshiah V, Divakar H, Gupte S, Datta M, Kapur A, Balaji V. Need for testing glucose tolerance in the early weeks of pregnancy. Indian Journal of Endocrinology and Metabolism. 2016;**20**:43-46

[31] Jimennez MoLeon J, Bueno-Cavanillas A, Luna-Del-Castillo JD, et al. Predictive value of screen for GD, influence of associated risk factors. Acta Obstetricia et Gynecologica Scandinavica. 2000;**79**:991-998

[32] Ahkter J, Qureshi R, Rahim F, et al. Diabetes in pregnancy in Pakistani women: Prevalence and complications in an indigenous south Asian community diabetic African health sciences, Vol. 4(1); 14 April 2004. Medicine. 1996;**13**(3):189-191

[33] Bancrofti K, Tuffnel DJ, Mason GC, et al. A randomised controlled pilot study for the management of gestational impaired glucose tolerance. BJOG: An International Journal of Obstetrics and Gynaecology. 2000;**107**:959-963

[34] Young C, Kuehl TJ, Sulak PJ, Allen RS. GD screening in subsequent pregnancy of previously healthy patients. American Journal of Obstetrics and Gynecology. 2000;**181**(4):798-802

[35] Dornhost A, Pateson EM, Nicholls JSD, et al. High prevalence of GD in

women from ethnic minority groups. Diabetic Medicine. 1992;**9**:820-825

[36] King H. Epidemiology of glucose intolerance and GD in woman of child bearing age. Diabetes Care. 1998;**21**(Suppll.2):B9-B13

[37] Danilenko Dixon DR, Van-Winter JJ, Nelson RL, Ogbum PL, et al. Universal versus selective screening application of 1997 ADA recommendation. The Obstetrician and Gynaecologist. 1999;**181**(4):798-802

[38] WHO. Prevention of Diabetes Mellitus, WHO Technical Report Series 884; 1994

[39] O'Sulivan JB, Mahan CM, Charles D, et al. Screening criteria for high risk GD. American Journal of Obstetrics and Gynecology. 1973;**116**:895-896

[40] Pettitt DJ, Knowler WC, Baird HR, et al. Gestational diabetes: Infant and maternal complication of pregnancy in relation to third-trimester glucose tolerance in Pima Indians. Diabetes Care. 1980;**3**:458-464

[41] Naylor CD, Sermer M, Chen E, Sykora K. Caesarian delivery in relation to birth weight and glucose gestational tolerance. Journal of the American Medical Association. 1996;**275**(15):1164-1170

[42] Khaundelwal M, Homko C, Reece EA. Gestational diabetes: Controversial and current opinion. Current Opinion in Obstetrics and Gynecology. 1999;**11**(2):157-165

[43] Moses RG. The recurrence rate of GD in subsequent pregnancies. Diabetes Care. 1996;**19**:1348

[44] Moulsted-Pederson L, Skouby SV, Damm P. Preconception counseling and contraception after gestational diabetes. Diabetes. 1991;**40**(Suppl 2):147-150

[45] Kjos SL, Peters RK, Xiang A, et al. Predicting future diabetes in Latino women with GD. Diabetes. 1995;**44**:586-591

[46] James Schelesselman. Formula for Calculation of Sample Size for Comparative Studies; 1974

[47] WHO Consultation Report 1999 on Diagnosis and Classification of DM

[48] Siribaddana SH, Deshabandu R, Rajapakse D, et al. The prevalence of GD in Sri Lankan antenatal clinic. The Ceylon Medical Journal. 1998;**43**(2):88-91

[49] Solomon CG, Willet WC, Carey VJ, et al. A prospective study of pregravid determinants of GD. The Journal of the American Medical Association. 1997;**278**:1078

[50] Coustan D. Management of GD: A self-fulfilling prophecy? The Journal of the American Medical Association. 1996;**275**:895-900

[51] Enkin M, Keirse MJ, Nelson J, et al. Gestational diabetes. In: A Guide to Effective Care in Pregnancy and Childbirth. Oxford University Press; 2000. pp. 75-78

[52] Jovanovic L. Screening, diagnosis, treatment and course of GD. UpToDate. 2002;**10**(1):93-107

[53] Ye J, Zhang L, Chen Y, Fang F, Luo Z, Zhang J. Searching for the definition of macrosomia through an outcome-based approach. PLoS One. 2014;**9**(6):e100192

[54] World Health Organisation. Diagnostic Criteria and Classification of Hyperglycaemia First Detected in Pregnancy. 2013. Available from: http://www.who.int/en/ [Accessed: January 15, 2015]

[55] Nankervis A, McIntyre H, Moses R, Ross G, Callaway L, Porter C, et al. ADIPS Consensus Guidelines for the

Testing and Diagnosis of Gestational Diabetes in Australia and New Zealand. 2014. Available from: http://adips.org/ [Accessed: January 15, 2015]

[56] Tieu J, McPhee A, Crowther C, Middleton P. Screening and subsequent management for gestational diabetes for improving maternal and infant health. Cochrane Database of Systematic Reviews. 2014;(2):CD007222. DOI: 10.1002/14651858.CD007222.pub3.2014

[57] Department of Health Queensland. GD Data 2006-2013. Perinatal Data Collection, Health Statistics Branch; 2014

[58] Australian Institute of Health and Welfare. Diabetes in Pregnancy: Its Impact on Australian Women and Their Babies. Diabetes Series No. 14. Cat. No. CVD 52. Canberra. 2010. Available from: http://www.aihw.gov.au [Accessed: December 05, 2014]

[59] Diabetes Australia Ltd. The National Diabetes Service Scheme (NDSS). 2015. Available from: http://www.ndss.com.au/ [Accessed: January 5, 2015]

[60] American Diabetes Association. Position statement: Standards of medical care in diabetes 2014. Diabetes Care. 2014;**37**(Supplement 1):S14-S80

[61] Queensland Health. Maternity services. In: Clinical Services Capability Framework for Public and Licensed Private Health Facilities v3.2. Brisbane: Queensland Government Department of Health; 2012. Available from: http://www.health.qld.gov.au

[62] Australian Commission on Safety and Quality in Healthcare. National Consensus Statement: Essential Elements for Recognising and Responding to Clinical Deterioration. 2010. Available from: http://www.safetyandquality.gov.au/ [Accessed: May 14, 2014]

[63] Willcox JC, Campbell KJ, van der Pligt P, Hoban E, Pidd D, Wilkinson S. Excess gestational weight gain: An exploration of midwives' views and practice. BMC Pregnancy and Childbirth. 2012;**12**:102

[64] Blumer I, Hadar E, Hadden DR, Jovanovic L, Mestman JH, Hassan Murad M, et al. Diabetes and pregnancy: An Endocrine Society clinical practice guideline. The Journal of Clinical Endocrinology and Metabolism. 2013;**98**:4227-4249

[65] Falavigna M, Schmidt MI, Trujillo J, Alves LF, Wendland ER, Torloni MR, et al. Effectiveness of gestational diabetes treatment: A systematic review with quality of evidence assessment. Diabetes Research and Clinical Practice. 2012;**98**(3):396-405

[66] Hartling L, Dryden DM, Guthrie A, Muise M, Vandermeer B, Donovan L. Benefits and harms of treating gestational diabetes: A systematic review and meta-analysis for the U.S. preventive services task force and the National Institutes of Health Office of medical applications of research. Annals of Internal Medicine. 2013;**159**(2):123-129

[67] Landon MB, Spong CY, Thom E, Carpenter MW, Ramin SM, Casey B, et al. A multicenter, randomized trial of treatment for mild gestational diabetes. The New England Journal of Medicine. 2009;**361**(14):1339-1348

[68] Australian Health Ministers' Advisory Council. Clinical Practice Guidelines: Antenatal Care-Module II. Canberra: Australian Government Department of Health. 2014. Available from: http://www.health.gov.au/antental [Accessed: January 15, 2015]

[69] Rauh-Hain JA, Rana S, Tamez H, Wang A, Cohen B, Cohen A, et al. Risk for developing gestational diabetes in women with twin pregnancies. The Journal of Maternal-Fetal & Neonatal Medicine. 2009;**22**(4):293-299

[70] Han S, Crowther C, Middleton P. Interventions for pregnant women with hyperglycaemia not meeting gestational diabetes and type 2 diabetes diagnostic criteria. Cochrane Database of Systematic Reviews. 2012;**1**:CD009037. DOI: 10.1002/14651858.CD009037.pub2.2012

[71] Wendland EM, Torloni MR, Falavigna M, Trujillo J, Dode MA, Campos MA, et al. Gestational diabetes and pregnancy outcomes-a systematic review of the World Health Organization (WHO) and the International Association of Diabetes in pregnancy study groups (IADPSG) diagnostic criteria. BMC Pregnancy and Childbirth. 2012;**12**:23

[72] Schmidt MI, Duncan BB, Reichelt AJ, Branchtein L, Matos MC, Costa e Forti A, et al. Gestational diabetes diagnosed with a 2-h 75-g oral glucose tolerance test and adverse pregnancy outcomes. Diabetes Care. 2001;**24**(7):1151-1155

[73] MacNeill S, Dodds L, Hamilton DC, Armson BA, VandenHof M. Rates and risk factors for recurrence of gestational diabetes. Diabetes Care. 2001;**24**(4):659-662

[74] Metzger BE, Buchanan TA, Coustan DR, de Leiva A, Dunger DB, Hadden DR, et al. Summary and recommendations of the fifth international workshop-conference on gestational diabetes. Diabetes Care. 2007;**30**(Suppl 2):S251-S260

[75] Agency for Healthcare Research and Quality. Gestational diabetes: Caring for women during and after pregnancy. Publication No.09-EHC014-3. Queensland Clinical Guideline: Gestational Diabetes Refer to Online Version, Destroy Printed Copies After Use Page 33 of 38; 2009

[76] Malcolm JC, Lawson ML, Gaboury I, Lough G, Keely E. Glucose tolerance of offspring of mother with gestational diabetes in a low-risk population. Diabetic Medicine. 2005;**23**:565-570

[77] Oostdam N, van Poppel MN, Wouters MG, van Mechelen W. Interventions for preventing gestational diabetes: A systematic review and meta-analysis. Journal of Women's Health. 2011;**20**(10):1551-1563

[78] Laitinen K, Poussa T, Isolauri E. Probiotics and dietary counselling contribute to glucose regulation during and after pregnancy: A randomised controlled trial. The British Journal of Nutrition. 2009;**101**(11):1679-1687

[79] Paxton G, Teale G, Nowson C, Mason R, McGrath J, Thompson M, et al. Vitamin D and health in pregnancy, infants, children and adolescents in Australia and New Zealand: A position statement. The Medical Journal of Australia. 2013;**198**(3):1-8

[80] Barakat R, Pelaez M, Lopez C, Lucia A, Ruiz JR. Exercise during pregnancy and gestational diabetes-related adverse effects: A randomised controlled trial. British Journal of Sports Medicine. 2013;**47**(10):630-636

[81] Nobles C, Marcus BH, Stanek EJ 3rd, Braun B, Whitcomb BW, Solomon CG, et al. Effect of an exercise intervention on gestational diabetes: A randomized controlled trial. Obstetrics and Gynecology. 2015;**125**(5):1195-1204

[82] Russo LM, Nobles C, Ertel KA, Chasan-Taber L, Whitcomb BW. Physical activity interventions in pregnancy and risk of gestational diabetes. Obstetrics and Gynecology. 2015;**125**(3):576-582

[83] Thangaratinam S, Rogozinska E, Jolly K, Glinkowski S, Duda W, Borowiack E, et al. Interventions to reduce or prevent obesity in pregnant women: A systematic review. Health Technology Assessment. 2012;**16**(31):1-191

[84] Tobias D, Zhang C, van Dam R, Bower K, Hu F. Physical activity before and during pregnancy and risk of gestational diabetes. Diabetes Care. 2011;**34**:223-229

[85] Humulin R. U-100 Package Insert. Indianapolis, Indiana: Eli Lilly and Company; 2015

[86] Zuckerwise LC, Werner EF, Pettker CM, McMahon-Brown EK, Thung SS, Han C. Pregestational diabetes with extreme insulin resistance: Use of U-500 insulin in pregnancy. Obstetrics and Gynecology. 2012;**120**:439-442

[87] Humulin R. U-500 Package Insert. Indianapolis, Indiana: Eli Lilly and Company; 2014

[88] NovoLog. Package Insert. Bagsvaerd, Denmark: Novo Nordisk; 2015

[89] Mathiesen ER, Kinsley B, Amiel SA, et al. Maternal glycemic control and hypoglycemia in type 1 diabetic pregnancy: A randomized trial of insulin aspart versus human insulin in 322 pregnant women. Diabetes Care. 2007;**30**:771-776

[90] Humalog. Package Insert. Indianapolis, Indiana: Eli Lilly and Company; 2015

[91] Apidra. Package Insert. Bridgewater, NJ: Sanofi-Aventis; 2015

[92] Humulin N. Package Insert. Indianapolis, Indiana: Eli Lilly and Company; 2015

[93] Levemir. Package Insert. Bagsvaerd, Denmark: Novo Nordisk; 2015

[94] Herrera KM, Rosenn BM, Foroutan J, et al. Randomized controlled trial of insulin detemir versus NPH for the treatment of pregnant women with diabetes. American Journal of Obstetrics and Gynecology. 2015;**213**:426.e1-4426e7

[95] Schnedl WJ, Krause R, Halwachs-Baumann G, Trinker M, Lipp RW, Krejs GJ. Evaluation of HbA1c determination methods in patients with hemoglobinopathies. Diabetes Care. 2000;**23**(3):339-344

[96] Monami M, Luzzi C, Lamanna C, Chiasserini V, Addante F, Desideri CM, et al. Three-year mortality in diabetic patients treated with different combinations of insulin secretagogues and metformin. Diabetes/Metabolism Research and Reviews. 2006;**22**(6):477-482

[97] Gidwani S. Solid Oral Dosage Form of Metformin and Glyburide and the Method of Preparation Thereof. U.S. Patent US20040175421, 2004

[98] de Veciana M, Major CA, Morgan MA, Asrat T, Toohey JS, Lien JM, et al. Postprandial versus preprandial blood glucose monitoring in women with gestational diabetes mellitus requiring insulin therapy. The New England Journal of Medicine. 1995;**333**:1237-1241

[99] Buchanan TA, Kjos SL, Montoro MN, Wu PYK, Madrilejo NG, Gonzalez M, et al. Use of fetal ultrasound to select metabolic therapy for pregnancies complicated by mild gestational diabetes. Diabetes Care. 1994;**17**:275-283

[100] Kjos SL, Schaefer-Graf U, Sardesi S, Peters RK, Buley A, Xiang AH, et al. A randomized controlled trial utilizing glycemic plus fetal ultrasound parameters versus glycemic parameters to determine insulin therapy in gestational diabetes with fasting hyperglycemia. Diabetes Care. 2001;**24**:1904-1910

[101] Zhu WW, Yang HX, Wei YM, Yan J, Wang ZL, Li XL, et al. Evaluation of the value of fasting plasma glucose

in the first prenatal visit to diagnose gestational diabetes in China. Diabetes Care. 2013;**36**(3):586-590

[102] Hughes RC, Moore MP, Gullam JE, Mohamed K, Rowan J. An early pregnancy HbA1c >/=5.9% (41 mmol/Mol) is optimal for detecting diabetes and identifies women at increased risk of adverse pregnancy outcomes. Diabetes Care. 2014;**37**(11):2953-2959

[103] Balaji V, Madhuri BS, Ashalatha S, Sheela S, Suresh S, Seshiah V. A1C in gestational diabetes in Asian Indian women. Diabetes Care. 2007;**30**(7):1865-1867

[104] Fong A, Serra AE, Gabby L, Wing DA, Berkowitz KM. Use of hemoglobin A1c as an early predictor of gestational diabetes. American Journal of Obstetrics and Gynecology. 2014;**21**(641):e1-e7

[105] Jones GR, Barker G, Goodall I, Schneider HG, Shephard MD, Twigg SM. Change of HbA1c reporting to the new SI units. The Medical Journal of Australia. 2011;**195**(1):45-46

[106] Crowther CA, Hiller JE, Moss JR, McPhee AJ, Jeffries WS, Robinson JS. Effect of treatment of gestational diabetes on pregnancy outcomes. The New England Journal of Medicine. 2005;**352**(24):2477-2486

[107] East C, Dolan W, Forster D. Antenatal breast milk expression by women with diabetes for improving infant outcomes. Cochrane Database of Systematic Reviews. 2014;**7**:CD010408. DOI: 10.1002/14651858.CD010408.pub2.2014

[108] Forster DA, Jacobs S, Amir LH, Davis P, Walker SP, McEgan K, et al. Safety and efficacy of antenatal milk expressing for women with diabetes in pregnancy: Protocol for a randomised controlled trial. BMJ Open. 2014;**4**(10):e006571

[109] Soltani H, Scott AM. Antenatal breast expression in women with diabetes: Outcomes from a retrospective cohort study. International Breastfeeding Journal. 2012;**7**(1):18

[110] Ismail NAM, Raji HO, Wahab AN, Mustafa N, Kamaruddin NA, Jamil MA. Glycemic control among pregnant diabetic women on insulin who fasted during ramadan. Iranian Journal of Medical Sciences. 2011;**36**(4):254-259

[111] Black MH, Sacks DA, Xiang AH, Lawrence JM. The relative contribution of prepregnancy overweight and obesity, gestational weight gain, and IADPSG-defined gestational diabetes to fetal overgrowth. Diabetes Care. 2013;**36**(1):56-62 Available from: mdc

[112] Institute of Medicine. Weight Gain During Pregnancy. Reexamining the Guidelines. 2009. Available from: www.iom.edu [Accessed: December 05, 2014]

[113] Queensland Clinical Guidelines. Obesity in Pregnancy. Guideline No. MN15.14-V5-R20. Queensland Health. 2015. Available from: http://www.health.qld.gov.au/qcg/

Section 2

Management

Chapter 3

Treatment of Gestational Diabetes

Ahmed Mohamed Maged

Abstract

Management of gestational diabetes mellitus (GDM) should consider both the maternal, fetal, and neonatal effects of the disease, line of treatment, and physiological changes during pregnancy. Women with GDM are classified into two categories according to their fasting blood glucose levels. Dietary control is mandatory in both classes, and the addition of pharmacological agents in those with fasting and 2-h postprandial plasma glucose levels <95 and 120 mg/dL is controversial (American College of Obstetricians and Gynecologists, 2013). Individualization of the diet in GDM according to women weight and height is recommended by the American Diabetes Association (ADA), and restriction of carbohydrate to a level that maintains normal glucose level is mandatory with individualization of the caloric intake according to women BMI and weight gain during pregnancy.

Keywords: gestational diabetes, management, diabetic diet, insulin, exercise, oral hypoglycemic

1. Introduction

The main aim of treatment of gestational diabetes is to prevent fetal, maternal, and neonatal complications. A randomized controlled trial which involved 1000 women with GDM showed that treatment of GDM is associated with the reduction of all neonatal complications, namely, birth injuries, shoulder dystocia, and perinatal morbidity and mortality. Treatment also reduced the rate of development of preeclampsia from 18 to 12% and the rate of large for gestational age (LGA) from 22 to 13% [1]. Even in women with mild GDM, treatment reduced the rate of LGA, the mass of neonatal fat, shoulder dystocia, cesarean section, and hypertensive disorders associating pregnancy [2, 3].

Improving the pregnancy outcome in women with GDM can be achieved through maintenance of fasting blood sugar levels <95 mg/dl (5.3 mmol/L), 1-h postprandial blood sugar <140 mg/dl (7.8 mmol/L), and 2-h postprandial blood sugar <120 mg/dl as recommended by both the American College of Obstetricians and Gynecologists (ACOG) and American Diabetes Association [4].

The treatment of GDM starts with dietary modifications along with particular nutritional approaches [5–7] combined with exercise [8, 9]. If this combination failed to maintain the needed glucose levels, pharmacological treatment starts, regardless of the lines used for treatment, proper monitoring of maternal health, fetal condition, and blood sugar levels.

1.1 Dietary modifications

Dietary counseling should be individualized according to women weight and height [10] through a registered dietitian [11].

 IntechOpen

JSOG committee on nutrient and metabolism problems described a caloric intake of 25–30 kcal/kg (+150 Kcal for the first half and + 350 kcal for the second half of pregnancy) [12].

The Ministry of Health and Welfare recommended a caloric intake of 25–30 kcal/kg (+ 50,250 and 450 kcal for the first, second, and third trimester, respectively) [13].

The ideal diet components are not yet determined. However excessive weight gain with postprandial hyperglycemia is commonly associated with diet that included 50–60% of carbohydrate. ACOG recommended the limitation of carbohydrate to 33–40% of the required calories and the remaining 60% to be gained from proteins (20%) and fats (40%) [4].

The complex form of carbohydrates is preferable over simple ones as they are absorbed slower without producing significant hyperglycemia. Complex carbohydrates also decrease insulin resistance [6].

If the routine three meals daily failed to achieve the target blood sugar, each meal should be divided in 2:1 or 1:1 ratio to eat 4–6 meals per day [14].

The ADA recommended "MyPlate" as a healthy guide for each meal which consists of 25% protein, 25% starch, and 50% non-starchy foods as vegetables especially steamed ones. Creating MyPlate is a simple and effective method allowing proper control of the blood glucose levels and losing weight (http://www.diabetes.org/food-and-fitness/food/planning-meals/create-your-plate/).

Some foods to be avoided include highly processed foods as white bread, fast foods, alcohol, baked products as muffins and cakes, sugary drinks, candy, and high starch foods as white rice and white potatoes.

2. Exercise

Although there are many randomized studies done to evaluate the effects of physical exercise and lifestyle modifications in adults with diabetes, only few ones evaluated these effects in pregnant women with GDM. These studies proved that exercise improves the blood glucose [8, 15–18]. These beneficial effects may occur as a result of the increase of lean muscle mass with subsequent increase in insulin sensitivity. So a moderate exercise program is highly recommended for women with GDM [11]. A moderate intensity aerobic exercise for at least 150 minutes weekly [19] or simple exercise as walking after each meal for 10–15 minutes [20] is recommended.

The Finnish GDM prevention trial (RADIEL)—a multicenter randomized controlled study—evaluated the efficacy of combined dietary and physical activity modifications in prevention of GDM and obesity-related perinatal complications [21]. Counseling was achieved through three visits to the study nurse at 13, 23, and 35 weeks of pregnancy. Dietary modification was done according to Nordic Nutrition Recommendations encouraging the intake of vegetables, fruits and berries, high-fiber whole-grain products, low-fat dairy products, vegetable fats high in unsaturated fatty acids, and fish and low-fat meat products with lower intake of sugar- and saturated fatty acid-rich foods. [22]. Physical moderate exercise for 150 minutes at least per week is recommended [23]. They found that these modifications had no effects on either the incidence of GDM or perinatal complications [24].

2.1 Pharmacologic treatment

Pharmacologic treatment is indicated when dietary management and exercise failed to achieve the target glucose levels.

Basically, insulin is the standard treatment for GDM [11]. Insulin has the advantage of non-crossing of the placenta. It is given according to the timing of the occurrence of hyperglycemia. If hyperglycemia is present throughout the day both in the fasting and postprandial state, a divided dose of combination of either long or intermediate acting insulin with the short acting one is recommended. The typical total starting dose is 0.7–1 unit/ kg of body weight. If hyperglycemia is detected only at a specific times, focusing the insulin dose at that specific time of hyperglycemia is done, e.g., high fasting blood sugar is treated using a nighttime intermediate-acting insulin, while elevated post-breakfast blood sugar is treated by short-acting insulin before breakfast. The maintenance dose is then adjusted according to the monitored blood glucose [4].

The insulin analogs as insulin aspart and lispro are preferred over the regular insulin as a short-acting type. They do not cross the placenta, and their main advantage is their faster onset of action allowing the women to receive their injection at the time of the meal not 10–15 minutes before it as needed in the regular type. This advantage provides better control of the glucose level, and less attacks of hypoglycemia resulted from timing error [25, 26]. Intermediate- and long-acting insulin include the basic isophane insulin (NPH) and recent insulin glargine and detemir (**Table 1**) [27–29].

2.1.1 Oral antidiabetic medications

Historically oral hypoglycemics should be avoided as early agents cross the placenta, resulting in fetal hyperinsulinemia with subsequent macrosomia and congenital malformations (most commonly in the ear) and severe neonatal hypoglycemia. Now their use in GDM is increasing despite them not approved by the US Food and Drug Administration [31] and the recommendation of ADA that insulin is the first-line therapy for GDM [11] as these products have advantages as ease of tablet intake, ease of storage, and safe needle disposal.

Oral antidiabetic medications include biguanides, sulfonylurea, acarbose, Guar gum, and thiazolidinedione.

Metformin is a biguanide that decreases intestinal glucose absorption and hepatic gluconeogenesis and increases peripheral glucose uptake. Historically, it was given to women used in pregestational diabetic women and women with polycystic ovary syndrome who suffer from infertility. In the latter group, it was continued until completion of the first trimester, despite the limited evidence of its ability to improve pregnancy outcome [32].

Type	Onset (min)	Peak (h)	Duration (h)
Insulin lispro	1–15	1–2	4–5
Insulin aspart	1–15	1–2	4–5
Regular insulin	30–60	2–4	6–8
Isophane insulin suspension (NPH)	60–180	5–7	13–18
Insulin glargine	60–120	No peak	24
Insulin detemir	60–180	Minimal at 8–10	18–26

Modified from Gabbe and Graves [30].

Table 1.
Describes the onset, peak, and duration of action of the commonly used insulins.

Although metformin can cross the placenta, its long-term metabolic effects on the growing fetus are not known [33]. One study showed the absence of any developmental effects till the age of 2 years of life [34].

In a randomized controlled trial, 751 pregnant women having GDM were assigned to treatment with insulin or metformin ± insulin. The perinatal outcome was similar among the two groups [35].

Another smaller trial showed that women assigned to metformin had lower blood glucose, lower maternal weight gain during pregnancy, and lower incidence of neonatal hypoglycemia [36].

In a network meta-analysis that included unpublished trials, there was a difference between insulin and metformin treatments regarding neonatal birth weight, hypoglycemia, or mode of delivery [37].

Therefore, women with GDM are carefully counseled about the use of metformin. They should know that it is not superior to insulin, there are no definitive data about its long-term effects of the growing fetus, and 26–46% of women on metformin will need to add insulin to replace it or to potentiate its effects for better glucose control [35, 36].

Metformin starting dose is usually 500 mg once daily at nighttime for 1 week, and then the dose is increased according to the response. The maximum daily dose is 2500–3000 mg daily in two–three divided doses.

Contraindications to metformin include impaired kidney function, and serum creatinine should be evaluated before the start of treatment.

Side effects of metformin occur in 2.5–45.7% of cases [38], and the commonest is GIT upset in the form of abdominal pain and diarrhea. Its use may be associated with higher rate of lactic acidosis, preeclampsia, and neonatal jaundice. So the drug is instructed to be administered with meals and to increase the needed dose gradually.

A systematic review stated that metformin use during pregnancy is safe and effective regarding the short-term pregnancy outcomes. There are no solid guidelines about the duration of metformin use during pregnancy, so it is based on clinical experience on a case-by-case basis [39].

Sulfonylurea used in GDM includes glyburide, tolbutamide, glibenclamide, and gliclazide. Chlorpropamide crosses, while glibenclamide does not cross the placenta.

Glyburide augments insulin secretion by pancreas (through binding adenosine triphosphate potassium channel receptors of the beta cells) and extrapancreatic tissues. It also increases insulin sensitivity of peripheral tissues. It should not be used as a first-line treatment as most studies showed inferior results when compared to insulin or metformin [31].

The dose of glyburide is 2.5–20 mg per day in divided doses. The maximum dose is 30 mg daily [40]. Even with these high doses, 4–16% of patients will need the addition of insulin for adequate glycemic control [41–44].

Contraindications include allergy to sulfa, and side effects include mild infrequent GIT side effects as nausea, vomiting, and diarrhea.

Although some individual trials showed no difference regarding blood glucose control between glyburide and insulin [41–46], meta-analyses reported higher incidence of macrosomia, maternal, and neonatal hypoglycemia [35, 36, 47]. Other trials found that women used glyburide and had higher incidence of hypertension, hyperbilirubinemia, and still birth than those on insulin therapy [31, 42, 48–52].

Other sulfonylurea include Thiazolidinedione as Pioglitazone & Rosiglitazone which decrease insulin resistance by reducing RESISTIN hormone released from adipose tissue. Their use during pregnancy cannot be recommended as no enough reports to support their use.

A Cochrane meta-analysis evaluated 7381 women with GDM and reported similar pregnancy outcomes when insulin therapy is compared with oral antidiabetic agents (metformin, glyburide, both, and acarbose) [53]. However these oral antidiabetic agents have different safety and efficacy, so pooling all of them together against insulin weakens that meta-analysis.

To sum up, the current available data show the absence of short-term hazards, but the long-term effects are still unknown. So, the women should be counseled about the unknown proven safety of the oral antidiabetic agents and the high rate of need for adding insulin before describing it.

ACOG considers insulin as the first-line treatment for GDM and describes oral agents (mainly metformin and rarely glyburide) as an alternative in women who decline insulin use (for financial issues or non-availability of safe administration) after proper consultation.

3. Other medications used in GDM

As there are many evidences that link oxidative stress and development of complications of diabetes with pregnancy, the use of antioxidants was suggested to improve pregnancy outcome [54]. Oxygen free radicals released during aerobic metabolism cause cellular damage [55, 56]. Many authors reported the participation of reactive oxygen species in diabetes associated with pregnancy [57, 58].

An interesting randomized controlled trial was conducted that involved 200 women with GDM who were assigned to receive antioxidant (1 gram L-ascorbic acid daily) or placebo. Maged and colleagues found that antioxidants significantly decreased the required insulin dose to control blood sugar and oxidative markers (glutathione, malondialdehyde, superoxide dismutase). In placental tissue homogenate, maternal blood and neonatal blood were significantly different between the two groups. In the antioxidant group, the neonatal blood sugar was more stable within 2 h of delivery, and the neonatal ICU admission was lower than other women. They concluded that the use of antioxidant administration during pregnancy in women with GDM reverses the oxidative stresses resulting in the improvement of neonatal outcome [59].

4. Glucose monitoring

Monitoring of glucose control is through blood testing urine analysis for glucose and ketone bodies and glycosylated hemoglobin.

The optimal frequency of blood glucose testing in women with GDM is not known. However, four evaluations daily seem to be satisfactory (fasting and after each meal) [4].

Fasting blood sugar is predictive of neonatal fat mass and subsequent development of childhood obesity and diabetes [60], and 1-h postprandial level was predictive of better blood sugar control and subsequent development of LGA and cesarean delivery [61], so both should be measured. The postprandial measurement can be after 1 or 2 h as the peak glucose level occurs almost 90 min after meals [62]. Measurement neither at 1 h nor at 2 h is superior to the other [63–65].

After stabilization of the blood sugar, individualization of the frequency of glucose measurement according to the gestational age, adherence of the patient to treatment and the needs of further adjustment is recommended. However the minimum is two measurements per day [4].

Women under self-monitoring of blood glucose daily had significantly lower incidence of fetal macrosomia and less weight gain than those under intermittent measurement of fasting glucose during semi-weekly antenatal visits [66].

de Veciana and colleagues randomly assigned 66 women with GDM for preprandial or 1-h postprandial measurement of blood sugar. They found that postprandial group had better blood glucose control with less macrosomia, cesarean delivery for cephalopelvic disproportion, and neonatal hypoglycemia [61].

A review included 10 trials of 538 women (468 and 70 women with type 1 and type 2 diabetes). Different glucose monitoring methods were compared without clear advantage of one method over the others. Two trials (43 women) comparing **self-monitoring versus standard care** proved no difference for cesarean section or glycemic control. One study (100 women) compared **self-monitoring versus hospitalization** and found no clear difference for hypertensive disorders, cesarean section, or preterm birth. Another study (61 women) which compared **preprandial versus postprandial glucose monitoring** proved no clear difference regarding cesarean section, macrosomia, or glycemic control. Three studies (84 women) which compared **automated telemedicine monitoring versus conventional system** found no clear difference for cesarean section and mortality or morbidity. **CGM was compared to intermittent monitoring** in two studies (225 women), and there was no difference for preeclampsia and cesarean section and large for gestational age. One trial (25 women) compared **constant CGM versus intermittent CGM** and found no clear difference between groups for cesarean section, glycemic control, or preterm birth [67].

4.1 Glycosylated hemoglobin

Hemoglobin (Hb) A forms about 90% of hemoglobin in adults, and its glycosylation occurs due to irreversible nonenzymatic binding of glucose to N-terminal of β chain. Hb A_1 is divided into Hb $A_{1\,a1}$, Hb $A_{1\,a2}$, Hb $A_{1\,b}$, and Hb $A_{1\,C}$ (the most important). The mean plasma glucose over the erythrocyte life span is correlated with the degree of glycosylation. Its advantages include that it is a single, non-fluctuating blood test that reflects the glucose levels over the last 4–8 weeks. So, HbA1c is an attractive test that can be added to routine investigations done in the first antenatal evaluation as it serves as a diagnostic tool for women with undiagnosed diabetes or at risk of its development [68]. If measured during the first trimester, it gives an idea about blood glucose control in the periconceptional period and during organogenesis. Its main disadvantage is its affection by red blood cell turnover [6] which results in the absence of clear recommendations for its use to diagnose GDM [69–71]. HbA1C increases also in cases of non-hemolytic anemias and chronic renal failure [72]. Women with A1c of 10–12% have up to a 25% risk of major malformations.

4.2 Fetal assessment

Like women with pregestational diabetes, women with GDM should follow antenatal fetal assessment especially those with poor glycemic control and women under medical treatment with insulin or oral antidiabetic agents [73]. It should start at 32 weeks of gestational age and earlier in women with GDM associated with other factors that may adversely affect fetal outcome as hypertensive disorders [74].

There is no consensus about antepartum fetal monitoring in properly controlled women without medical treatment, and if done it usually starts to alter at 32 weeks. The specific test used and its frequency are dependent on the regional practice, but amniotic fluid measurement is probably included as polyhydramnios is commonly associated with fetal hyperglycemia [4].

At Parkland Hospital, women with GDM are routinely asked to count daily fetal kick especially during the third trimester, and women on insulin treatment are offered for hospital admission and CTG monitoring three times weekly [74].

5. Obstetrical management

Timing and management of delivery of women with GDM are dependent on glycemic control, fetal condition, and associated complications. Women with proper glycemic control without associated medical problems are followed up till term [75, 76].

A comparison was done between women with GDM who were subjected to labor induction at 38 weeks and those who were followed up till 41 weeks of gestation, which revealed similar CS rate and all other outcomes except the higher occurrence of neonatal hyperbilirubinemia in one study [77], lower incidence of LGA in another study [78], and lower incidence of shoulder dystocia in a third one [79] in the induction group. A more recent study found a lower rate of CS in the induction group [80]. So women with GDM using medications with proper control of blood sugar delivered better during the 39 weeks of gestation [4].

In women with poor control of their blood sugar, timing of delivery is determined by balancing the risk of prematurity and the ongoing risk of intrauterine fetal death. In general earlier delivery in women with good glycemic control is recommended [75, 76], but the clear guides for glycemic control and timing of delivery are absent [81]. In general delivery between the start of 37 weeks and the completion of 38 weeks appears appropriate, while delivery at 34 weeks till the completed 36 weeks should be attempted only in women with abnormal fetal well-being assessment and those with failed hospital control of blood sugar [4].

Ultrasound assessment of fetal size should be done in all women with GDM. However only 22% of fetuses diagnosed as LGA by ultrasound had macrosomia after birth [82]. To prevent one case of permanent brachial plexus injury, 588 and 962 CS should be performed for ultrasonographic estimated fetal weight of 4500 and 4000 gm, respectively [83, 84]. So women with GDM and macrosomic fetus should be counseled about the elective CS risks and benefits [85].

6. Postpartum evaluation

Women with GDM should be evaluated postpartum as 15–70% will develop diabetes later in life [86–90]. These women were estimated to have sevenfold increased risk of developing type 2 DM when compared to controls [91]. So, screening after 4–12 weeks of delivery is recommended to identify those with diabetes, impaired fasting glucose levels, or impaired glucose tolerance [11] (**Figure 1**).

ACOG practice bulletin No. 190: Gestational diabetes mellitus [4].

The Fifth International Workshop-Conference on Gestational Diabetes recommended that women with GDM undergo evaluation with a 75-g oral glucose tolerance test at 6–12 weeks postpartum [92]. These recommendations are shown in **Table 2**.

Women with GDM are at an increased risk for cardiovascular complications associated with dyslipidemia, hypertension, and abdominal obesity—the *metabolic syndrome* [74].

Kessous and colleagues found that women with GDM were 2.6 times more likely to be hospitalized for cardiovascular morbidity [93].

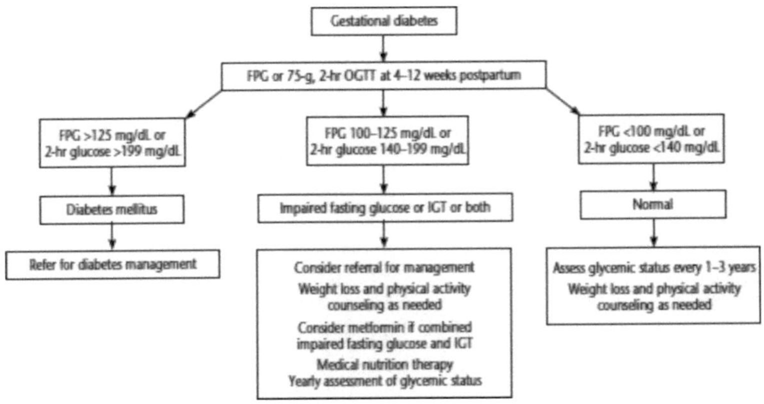

Figure 1.
Management of postpartum screening results. Abbreviations: FPG, fasting plasma glucose, OGTT, oral glucose tolerance test; IGT, impaired glucose tolerance.

Time	Test	Purpose
Post-delivery 1–3 days	Fasting or random plasma glucose	Detect persistent, overt diabetes
Early postpartum (6–12 week)	75 g, 2-h OGTT	Postpartum classification of glucose metabolism
1-year postpartum	75 g, 2-h OGTT	Assess glucose metabolism
Annually	Fasting plasma glucose	Assess glucose metabolism
Triannually	75 g, 2-h OGTT	Assess glucose metabolism
Prepregnancy	75 g, 2-h OGTT	Classify glucose metabolism

Metzger et al. [92].

Table 2.
Fifth international workshop-conference: Metabolic assessments recommended after pregnancy with gestational diabetes.

Shah and coworkers also reported excessive cardiovascular disease by 10 years in women with GDM [94].

7. Recurrent gestational diabetes

The risk of recurrence of GDM is estimated to be 40% in primiparous women [95]. Women with higher body mass index are more likely to have impaired glucose tolerance in subsequent pregnancies. Therefore, lifestyle modifications, including weight control and exercise between pregnancies, may prevent the recurrence of GDM [96]. Overweight and obese women in their first pregnancy will lower the risk of GDM, if they lose 2 or more units of their body mass index [97]. The risk of GDM in second pregnancy was 4.2% in women without GDM in their first pregnancy against 41.3 percent in those with a history of gestational diabetes in their first pregnancy [98].

8. Contraception

Women with recent GDM can use low-dose hormonal contraceptives safely as the rate of developing of diabetes is similar in oral contraceptive users and nonusers of any hormonal contraception [99]. Care should be taken in women at risk of cardiovascular diseases as obese, hypertensive, and dyslipidemic women with direction of the contraceptive choice toward a method without potential cardiovascular consequences as intrauterine device.

Studies were reviewed and evaluated for quality according to the method outlined by the US Preventive Services Task Force:

I Evidence obtained from at least one properly designed randomized controlled trial.

II-1 Evidence obtained from well-designed controlled trials without randomization.

II-2 Evidence obtained from well-designed cohort or case–control analytic studies, preferably from more than one center or research group.

II-3 Evidence obtained from multiple time series with or without the intervention. Dramatic results in uncontrolled experiments also could be regarded as this type of evidence.

III Opinions of respected authorities, based on clinical experience, descriptive studies, or reports of expert committees.

Author details

Ahmed Mohamed Maged
Kasr Alainy Hospital, Cairo University, Egypt

*Address all correspondence to: dr_ahmedmaged08@kasralainy.edu.eg

References

[1] Crowther CA, Hiller JE, Moss JR, McPhee AJ, Jeffries WS, Robinson JS. Effect of treatment of gestational diabetes mellitus on pregnancy outcomes. Australian Carbohydrate Intolerance Study in Pregnant Women (ACHOIS) Trial Group. The New England Journal of Medicine. 2005;**352**:2477-2486

[2] Landon MB, Spong CY, Thom E, Carpenter MW, Ramin SM, Casey B, et al. A multicenter, randomized trial of treatment for mild gestational diabetes. Eunice Kennedy Shriver National Institute of Child Health and Human Development Maternal-Fetal Medicine Units Network. The New England Journal of Medicine. 2009;**361**:1339-1348

[3] Hartling L, Dryden DM, Guthrie A, Muise M, Vandermeer B, Donovan L. Benefits and harms of treating gestational diabetes mellitus: A systematic review and meta-analysis for the U.S. Preventive Services Task Force and the National Institutes of Health Office of Medical Applications of Research. Annals of Internal Medicine. 2013;**159**:123-129

[4] Committee on Practice Bulletins—Obstetrics. ACOG practice bulletin No. 190: Gestational diabetes mellitus. Obstetrics and Gynecology. 2018;**131**(2):e49-e64. DOI: 10.1097/AOG.0000000000002501

[5] Han S, Middleton P, Shepherd E, Van Ryswyk E, Crowther CA. Different types of dietary advice for women with gestational diabetes mellitus. Cochrane Database of Systematic Reviews. 2017;(2):CD009275. (Meta-analysis)

[6] Moses RG, Barker M, Winter M, Petocz P, Brand-Miller JC. Can a low-glycemic index diet reduce the need for insulin in gestational diabetes mellitus? A randomized trial. Diabetes Care. 2009;**32**:996-1000

[7] Louie JC, Markovic TP, Perera N, Foote D, Petocz P, Ross GP, et al. Diabetes Care. 2011;**34**:2341-2346

[8] Ceysens G, Rouiller D, Boulvain M. Exercise for diabetic pregnant women. Cochrane Database of Systematic Reviews. 2006;(3):CD004225. (Meta-analysis)

[9] Barakat R, Pelaez M, Lopez C, Lucia A, Ruiz JR. Exercise during pregnancy and gestational diabetes related adverse effects: A randomised controlled trial. British Journal of Sports Medicine. 2013;**47**:630-636

[10] Bantle JP, Wylie-Rosett J, Albright AL, et al. Nutrition recommendations and interventions for diabetes. Diabetes Care. 2008;**31**(1 Suppl):S61

[11] American Diabetes Association. Management of diabetes in pregnancy. Diabetes Care. 2017;**40**:S114-S119

[12] Sugawa T. Proposed committee report on nutrient and metabolism problems: Management policy for gestational diabetes mellitus and pregnant women with diabetes complications. Acta Obstetrica et Gynaecologica Japonica. 1985;**37**:473-477. (in Japanese)

[13] Ministry of Health, Labour and Welfare. Dietary Reference Intakes for Japanese (2010 Edition). 2nd ed. Tokyo: First Printing; 2010. (in Japanese)

[14] Sugiyama T. Management of Gestational Diabetes Mellitus. JMAJ. 2011;**54**(5):293-300

[15] Jovanovic-Peterson L, Durak EP, Peterson CM. Randomized trial of diet versus diet plus cardiovascular

conditioning on glucose levels in gestational diabetes. American Journal of Obstetrics and Gynecology. 1989;**161**:415-419

[16] Bung P, Bung C, Artal R, Khodiguian N, Fallenstein F, Spatling L. Therapeutic exercise for insulin-requiring gestational diabetics: Effects on the fetus—Results of a randomized prospective longitudinal study. Journal of Perinatal Medicine. 1993;**21**:125-137

[17] Halse RE, Wallman KE, Newnham JP, Guelfi KJ. Homebased exercise training improves capillary glucose profile in women with gestational diabetes. Medicine and Science in Sports and Exercise. 2014;**46**:1702-1709

[18] Anjana RM, Sudha V, Lakshmipriya N, Anitha C, Unnikrishnan R, Bhavadharini B, et al. Physical activity patterns and gestational diabetes outcomes – The wings project. Diabetes Research and Clinical Practice. 2016;**116**:253-262

[19] American Diabetes Association. Standards of medical care in diabetes—2011. Diabetes Care. 2011;**34**(Suppl. 1):S11-S61

[20] Davenport MH, Mottola MF, McManus R, Gratton R. A walking intervention improves capillary glucose control in women with gestational diabetes mellitus: A pilot study. Applied Physiology, Nutrition, and Metabolism. 2008;**33**:511-517

[21] Rönö K, Stach-Lempinen B, Klemetti MM, Kaaja RJ, Pöyhönen-Alho M, Eriksson JG, et al. Prevention of gestational diabetes through lifestyle intervention: Study design and methods of a Finnish randomized controlled multicenter trial (RADIEL). BMC Pregnancy and Childbirth. 2014;**14**:70

[22] Becker W, Lyhne N, Pedersen A, Aro A, Fogelholm M, Þhórsdottir I, et al. Nordic nutrition recommendations 2004 – Integrating nutrition and physical activity. Scandinavian Journal of Nutrition. 2004;**48**:178-187

[23] ACOG Committee on Obstetric Practice. ACOG committee opinion. Exercise during pregnancy and the postpartum period. Number 267, January 2002. American College of Obstetricians and Gynecologists. International Journal of Gynecology & Obstetrics. 2002;**77**:79-81

[24] Rönö K, Grotenfelt NE, Klemetti MM, Stach-Lempinen B, Huvinen E, Meinilä J, et al. Effect of a lifestyle intervention during pregnancy-findings from the Finnish gestational diabetes prevention trial (RADIEL). Journal of Perinatology. 2018;**38**:1157-1164. DOI: 10.1038/s41372-018-0178-8

[25] Zinman B, Tildesley H, Chiasson JL, Tsui E, Strack T. Insulin lispro in CSII: Results of a double-blind crossover study [published erratum appears in Diabetes 1997;46:1239]. Diabetes. 1997;**46**:440-443

[26] Anderson JH Jr, Brunelle RL, Koivisto VA, Pfutzner A, Trautmann ME, Vignati L, et al. Reduction of postprandial hyperglycemia and frequency of hypoglycemia in IDDM patients on insulin-analog treatment. Multicenter insulin Lispro study group. Diabetes. 1997;**46**:265-270

[27] Herrera KM, Rosenn BM, Foroutan J, Bimson BE, Al Ibraheemi Z, Moshier EL, et al. Randomized controlled trial of insulin detemir versus NPH for the treatment of pregnant women with diabetes. American Journal of Obstetrics and Gynecology. 2015;**213**:426.e1-426.e7

[28] Koren R, Toledano Y, Hod M. The use of insulin detemir during pregnancy: A safety evaluation. Expert Opinion on Drug Safety. 2015;**14**:593-599

[29] Lv S, Wang J, Xu Y. Safety of insulin analogs during pregnancy: A meta-analysis. Archives of Gynecology and Obstetrics. 2015;**292**:749-756

[30] Gabbe SG, Graves CR. Management of diabetes mellitus complicating pregnancy. Obstetrics and Gynecology. 2003;**102**:857-868

[31] Camelo Castillo W, Boggess K, Sturmer T, Brookhart MA, Benjamin DK Jr, Jonsson FM. Trends in glyburide compared with insulin use for gestational diabetes treatment in the United States, 2000-2011. Obstetrics and Gynecology. 2014;**123**:1177-1184

[32] De Leo V, Musacchio MC, Piomboni P, Di Sabatino A, Morgante G. The administration of metformin during pregnancy reduces polycystic ovary syndrome related gestational complications. European Journal of Obstetrics, Gynecology, and Reproductive Biology. 2011;**157**:63-66

[33] Eyal S, Easterling TR, Carr D, Umans JG, Miodovnik M, Hankins GD, et al. Pharmacokinetics of metformin during pregnancy. Drug Metabolism and Disposition. 2010;**38**:833-840

[34] Wouldes TA, Battin M, Coat S, Rush EC, Hague WM, Rowan JA. Neurodevelopmental outcome at 2 years in offspring of women randomised to metformin or insulin treatment for gestational diabetes. Archives of Disease in Childhood. Fetal and Neonatal Edition. 2016;**101**:F488-F493

[35] Rowan JA, Hague WM, Gao W, Battin MR, Moore MP. Metformin versus insulin for the treatment of gestational diabetes. MiG trial investigators [published erratum appears in N Engl J Med 2008;359:106]. The New England Journal of Medicine. 2008;**358**:2003-2015

[36] Spaulonci CP, Bernardes LS, Trindade TC, Zugaib M, Francisco RP. Randomized trial of metformin vs insulin in the management of gestational diabetes. American Journal of Obstetrics and Gynecology. 2013;**209**:34.e1-7

[37] Farrar D, Simmonds M, Bryant M, Sheldon TA, Tuffnell D, Golder S, et al. Treatments for gestational diabetes: A systematic review and meta-analysis. BMJ Open. 2017;7:e015557. (Systematic Review and Meta-analysis)

[38] Balsells M, Garcia-Patterson A, Sola I, Roque M, Gich I, Corcoy R. Glibenclamide, metformin, and insulin for the treatment of gestational diabetes: A systematic review and meta-analysis. BMJ. 2015;**350**:h102. (Meta-analysis)

[39] Lautatzis ME, Goulis DG, Vrontakis M. Efficacy and safety of metformin during pregnancy in women with gestational diabetes mellitus or polycystic ovary syndrome: A systematic review. Metabolism. 2013 Nov;**62**(11):1522-1534. DOI: 10.1016/j.metabol.2013.06.006 Epub 2013 Jul 23

[40] Hebert MF, Ma X, Naraharisetti SB, Krudys KM, Umans JG, Hankins GD, et al. Are we optimizing gestational diabetes treatment with glyburide? The pharmacologic basis for better clinical practice. Obstetric-Fetal pharmacology research unit network. Clinical Pharmacology and Therapeutics. 2009;**85**:607-614

[41] Langer O, Conway DL, Berkus MD, Xenakis EM, Gonzales O. A comparison of glyburide and insulin in women with gestational diabetes mellitus. The New England Journal of Medicine. 2000;**343**:1134-1138

[42] Jacobson GF, Ramos GA, Ching JY, Kirby RS, Ferrara A, Field DR. Comparison of glyburide and insulin for the management of gestational diabetes in a large managed care organization. American Journal of Obstetrics and Gynecology. 2005;**193**:118-124

[43] Moore LE, Clokey D, Rappaport VJ, Curet LB. Metformin compared with glyburide in gestational diabetes: A randomized controlled trial. Obstetrics and Gynecology. 2010;**115**:55-59

[44] Camelo Castillo W, Boggess K, Sturmer T, Brookhart MA, Benjamin DK Jr, Jonsson FM. Association of adverse pregnancy outcomes with glyburide vs insulin in women with gestational diabetes. JAMA Pediatrics. 2015;**169**:452-458

[45] Anjalakshi C, Balaji V, Balaji MS, Seshiah V. A prospective study comparing insulin and glibenclamide in gestational diabetes mellitus in Asian Indian women. Diabetes Research and Clinical Practice. 2007;**76**:474-475

[46] Lain KY, Garabedian MJ, Daftary A, Jeyabalan A. Neonatal adiposity following maternal treatment of gestational diabetes with glyburide compared with insulin. American Journal of Obstetrics and Gynecology. 2009;**200**:501. e.16

[47] Song R, Chen L, Chen Y, Si X, Liu Y, Liu Y, et al. Comparison of glyburide and insulin in the management of gestational diabetes: A meta-analysis. PLoS One. 2017;**12**:e0182488. (Meta-analysis)

[48] Langer O, Yogev Y, Xenakis EM, Rosenn B. Insulin and glyburide therapy: Dosage, severity level of gestational diabetes, and pregnancy outcome. American Journal of Obstetrics and Gynecology. 2005;**192**:134-139

[49] Chmait R, Dinise T, Moore T. Prospective observational study to establish predictors of glyburide success in women with gestational diabetes mellitus. Journal of Perinatology. 2004;**24**:617-622

[50] Kahn SE, Haffner SM, Heise MA, Herman WH, Holman RR, Jones NP, et al. Glycemic durability of rosiglitazone, metformin, or glyburide monotherapy. ADOPT study group [published erratum appears in N Engl J Med 2007;356:1387-8]. The New England Journal of Medicine. 2006;**355**:2427-2443

[51] Rochon M, Rand L, Roth L, Gaddipati S. Glyburide for the management of gestational diabetes: Risk factors predictive of failure and associated pregnancy outcomes. American Journal of Obstetrics and Gynecology. 2006;**195**:1090-1094

[52] Cheng YW, Chung JH, Block-Kurbisch I, Inturrisi M, Caughey AB. Treatment of gestational diabetes mellitus: Glyburide compared to subcutaneous insulin therapy and associated perinatal outcomes. The Journal of Maternal-Fetal & Neonatal Medicine. 2012;**25**:379-384

[53] Brown J, Grzeskowiak L, Williamson K, Downie MR, Crowther CA. Insulin for the treatment of women with gestational diabetes. Cochrane Database of Systematic Reviews. 2017;(11):CD012037. (Systematic Review)

[54] Min J, Park B, Kim YJ, et al. Effect of oxidative stress on birth sizes: Consideration of window from mid pregnancy to delivery. Placenta. 2009;**30**:418-423

[55] Saugstad OD. Mechanisms of tissue injury by oxygen radicals: Implications for neonatal disease. Acta Paediatrica. 1996;**85**:1-4

[56] Halliwell B. Free radicals and antioxidants: A personal view. Nutrition Reviews. 1994;**52**:253-265

[57] Damasceno DC, Volpato GT, de MattosParanhos CI, Cunha Rudge MV. Oxidative stress and diabetes in pregnant rats. Animal Reproduction Science. 2002;**72**:235-244

[58] Brownlee M. The pathobiology of diabetic complications: A unifying mechanism. Diabetes. 2005;**54**:1615-1625

[59] Maged AM, Torky H, Fouad MA, GadAllah SH, Waked NM, Gayed AS, et al. Role of antioxidants in gestational diabetes mellitus and relation to fetal outcome: A randomized controlled trial. The Journal of Maternal-Fetal & Neonatal Medicine. 2016;**29**(24):4049-4054. DOI: 10.3109/14767058.2016.1154526

[60] Durnwald CP, Mele L, Spong CY, Ramin SM, Varner MW, Rouse DJ, et al. Glycemic characteristics and neonatal outcomes of women treated for mild gestational diabetes. Eunice Kennedy Shriver National Institute of Child Health and Human Development (NICHD) maternal-Fetal medicine units network (MFMU). Obstetrics and Gynecology. 2011;**117**:819-827

[61] de Veciana M, Major CA, Morgan MA, Asrat T, Toohey JS, Lien JM, et al. Postprandial versus preprandial blood glucose monitoring in women with gestational diabetes mellitus requiring insulin therapy. The New England Journal of Medicine. 1995;**333**:1237-1241

[62] Ben-Haroush A, Yogev Y, Chen R, Rosenn B, Hod M, Langer O. The postprandial glucose profile in the diabetic pregnancy. American Journal of Obstetrics and Gynecology. 2004;**191**:576-581

[63] Weisz B, Shrim A, Homko CJ, Schiff E, Epstein GS, Sivan E. One hour versus two hours postprandial glucose measurement in gestational diabetes: A prospective study. Journal of Perinatology. 2005;**25**:241-244

[64] Moses RG, Lucas EM, Knights S. Gestational diabetes mellitus. At what time should the postprandial glucose level be monitored? The Australian & New Zealand Journal of Obstetrics & Gynaecology. 1999;**39**:457-460

[65] Sivan E, Weisz B, Homko CJ, Reece EA, Schiff E. One or two hours postprandial glucose measurements: Are they the same? American Journal of Obstetrics and Gynecology. 2001;**185**:604-607

[66] Hawkins JS, Lo JY, Casey BM, et al. Diet-treated gestational diabetes: Comparison of early versus routine diagnosis. American Journal of Obstetrics and Gynecology. 2008;**198**:287

[67] Moy FM, Ray A, Buckley BS, West HM. Techniques of monitoring blood glucose during pregnancy for women with pre-existing diabetes. Cochrane Database of Systematic Reviews 11 Jun 2017;(6):CD009613. DOI: 10.1002/14651858.CD009613.pub3.

[68] Malkani S, Mordes JP. Implications of using hemoglobin A1C for diagnosing diabetes mellitus. The American Journal of Medicine. 2011;**124**:395-401

[69] Seino Y, Nanjo K, Tajima N, Kadowaki T, Kashiwagi A, Araki E, et al. Report of the committee on the classification and diagnostic criteria of diabetes mellitus. Journal of Diabetes Investigation. 2010;**1**:212-228

[70] Mosca A, Paleari R, Dalfra MG, Di Cianni G, Cuccuru I, Pellegrini G, et al. Reference intervals for hemoglobin A1c in pregnant women: Data from an Italian multicenter study. Clinical Chemistry. 2006;**52**:1138-1143

[71] Lowe LP, Metzger BE, Dyer AR, Lowe J, McCance DR, Lappin TR, et al. Hyperglycemia and adverse pregnancy outcome (HAPO) study: Associations of maternal A1C and glucose with pregnancy outcomes. Diabetes Care. 2012;**35**:574-580

[72] Benaiges D, Flores-Le Roux JA, Marcelo I, Mane L, Rodriguez M, Navarro X, et al. Is first-trimester HbA1c useful in the diagnosis of gestational diabetes? Diabetes Research and Clinical Practice. 2017;**133**:85-91

[73] Wu K, Cheng Y, Li T, Ma Z, Liu J, Zhang Q, et al. The utility of HbA1c combined with haematocrit for early screening of gestational diabetes mellitus. Diabetology and Metabolic Syndrome. *2018*;***10***:14 https://doi.org/10.1186/s13098-018-0314-9

[74] American College of Obstetricians and Gynecologists. Antepartum fetal surveillance. Practice bulletin No. 145. Obstetrics and Gynecology. 2014;**124**:182-192

[75] Cunningham FG, Leveno KJ, Bloom SL, et al. Diabetes mellitus. In: Cunningham FG, Williams JW, editors. William's Obstetrics. 24th ed. New York (NY): McGraw-Hill; 2014. pp. 1125-1146 [Chapter 57]

[76] Spong CY, Mercer BM, D'alton M, Kilpatrick S, Blackwell S, Saade G. Timing of indicated late-preterm and early-term birth. Obstetrics and Gynecology. 2011;**118**:323-333

[77] American College of Obstetricians and Gynecologists. Medically indicated late-preterm and early-term deliveries. Committee opinion No. 560. Obstetrics and Gynecology. 2013;**121**:908-910

[78] Alberico S, Erenbourg A, Hod M, Yogev Y, Hadar E, Neri F, et al. Immediate delivery or expectant management in gestational diabetes at term: The GINEXMAL randomised controlled trial. GINEXMAL group. BJOG. 2017;**124**:669-677

[79] Lurie S, Insler V, Hagay ZJ. Induction of labor at 38 to 39 weeks of gestation reduces the incidence of shoulder dystocia in gestational diabetic patients class A2. American Journal of Perinatology. 1996;**13**:293-296

[80] Witkop CT, Neale D, Wilson LM, Bass EB, Nicholson WK. Active compared with expectant delivery management in women with gestational diabetes: A systematic review. Obstetrics and Gynecology. 2009;**113**:206-217. (Systematic Review)

[81] Melamed N, Ray JG, Geary M, Bedard D, Yang C, Sprague A, et al. Induction of labor before 40 weeks is associated with lower rate of cesarean delivery in women with gestational diabetes mellitus. American Journal of Obstetrics and Gynecology. 2016;**214**:364.e1-8

[82] Caughey AB, Valent AM. When to deliver women with diabetes in pregnancy? American Journal of Perinatology. 2016;**33**:1250-1254

[83] Scifres CM, Feghali M, Dumont T, Althouse AD, Speer P, Caritis SN, et al. Large-for-gestational-age ultrasound diagnosis and risk for cesarean delivery in women with gestational diabetes mellitus. Obstetrics and Gynecology. 2015;**126**:978-986

[84] Rouse DJ, Owen J, Goldenberg RL, Cliver SP. The effectiveness and costs of elective cesarean delivery for fetal macrosomia diagnosed by ultrasound. JAMA. 1996;**276**:1480-1486

[85] Garabedian C, Deruelle P. Delivery (timing, route, peripartum glycemic control) in women with gestational diabetes mellitus. Diabetes & Metabolism. 2010;**36**:515-521

[86] American College of Obstetricians and Gynecologists. Fetal macrosomia. Practice bulletin No. 173. Obstetrics and Gynecology. 2016;**128**:e195-e209

[87] Kim C, Newton KM, Knopp RH. Gestational diabetes and the incidence of type 2 diabetes: A systematic review.

Diabetes Care. 2002;**25**:1862-1868. (Systematic Review)

[88] Kaaja RJ, Greer IA. Manifestations of chronic disease during pregnancy. JAMA. 2005;**294**:2751-2757

[89] Buchanan TA, Xiang AH. Gestational diabetes mellitus. The Journal of Clinical Investigation. 2005;**115**:485-491

[90] Russell MA, Phipps MG, Olson CL, Welch HG, Carpenter MW. Rates of postpartum glucose testing after gestational diabetes mellitus. Obstetrics and Gynecology. 2006;**108**:1456-1462

[91] Chodick G, Elchalal U, Sella T, Heymann AD, Porath A, Kokia E, et al. The risk of overt diabetes mellitus among women with gestational diabetes: A population-based study. Diabetic Medicine. 2010;**27**:779-785

[92] Bellamy L, Casas JP, Hingorani AD, Williams D. Type 2 diabetes mellitus after gestational diabetes: A systematic review and meta-analysis. Lancet. 2009;**373**:1773-1779. (Meta-analysis)

[93] Metzger BE, Buchanan TA, Coustan DR, et al. Summary and recommendations of the fifth international workshop-conference on gestational diabetes. Diabetes Care. 2007;**30**(Suppl 2):S251

[94] Kessous R, Shoham-Vardi I, Pariente G, et al. An association between gestational diabetes mellitus and long-term maternal cardiovascular morbidity. Heart. 2013;**99**:1118

[95] Shah BR, Retnakaran R, Booth GL. Increased risk of cardiovascular disease in young women following gestational diabetes. Diabetes Care. 2008;**31**(8):1668

[96] Holmes HJ, Casey BM, Lo JY, et al. Likelihood of diabetes recurrence in women with mild gestational diabetes (GDM). American Journal of Obstetrics and Gynecology. 2003;**189**(6):161

[97] Kim C, Cheng YJ, Beckles GL. Cardiovascular disease risk profiles in women with histories of gestational diabetes but without current diabetes. Obstetrics and Gynecology. 2008;**112**(4):875

[98] Ehrlich SF, Hedderson MM, Feng J, et al. Change in body mass index between pregnancies and the risk of gestational diabetes in a second pregnancy. Obstetrics and Gynecology. 2011;**117**(6):1323

[99] Getahun D, Fassett MJ, Jacobsen SJ. Gestational diabetes: Risk of recurrence in subsequent pregnancies. American Journal of Obstetrics and Gynecology. 2010;**203**:467

Chapter 4

Insulin Therapy in Gestational Diabetes

Anca Pantea-Stoian, Roxana Adriana Stoica and Simona Diana Stefan

Abstract

The prevalence of gestational diabetes risen in several populations during the past 20 years, and increased direct and indirect healthcare costs, including those for insulin treatment. Establishing the optimal treatment and initiation momentum are critical to achieve glycemic control and minimize the impact on fetal development and perinatal complications. Insulin is the only therapy that does not cross the placenta, and some of its types were proved to be safe in pregnancy. Intrapartum management is based on intravenous insulin administration, and standard protocols should be implemented in every center. Postpartum management requires special attention, as insulin necessary has a fast decline exposing mothers to hypoglycemia.

Keywords: gestational diabetes, insulin therapy, macrosomia, neonatal hypoglycemia

1. Introduction

Gestational diabetes (GD) is one of the most common pathologies in pregnancy. Gestational diabetes has been defined as any degree of glucose intolerance with onset or first recognition during pregnancy [1]. In pregnancy, there are multiple hormonal changes, including hyperinsulinemia and an insulin-resistant state; thus the pancreatic beta cell function becomes insufficient to meet the body's reasonable needs, and insulin must be injected.

There is also the possibility that hyperglycemia was present before the pregnancy; therefore International Association of Diabetes and Pregnancy Study Groups (IADPSG) defined the pregnancy hyperglycemia as either 'overt diabetes' or 'gestational diabetes mellitus' (GDM) [2].

Considering the ascending trend of type 2 diabetes mellitus and obesity from the last decades, GD has intuitively the same tendency [3, 4]. The prevalence of GD is estimated at approximately 135,000 cases per year in the US [5], representing on average 3–8% of all pregnancies [6]. It is estimated that the prevalence of GD has increased by 10–100% in several racial groups during the past 20 years, increasing direct and indirect healthcare costs [5].

The goal of treatment for women with GD (recommended by both American Diabetes Association-ADA, and the American College of Obstetricians and Gynecologists-ACOG) is a fasting plasma glucose level <95 mg/dl, a 1-hour post-prandial glucose level of less than 140 mg/dl and a 2-hour post-prandial glucose level of less than 120 mg/dl, whereas for the HbA1c the target is <6–6.5% (42–48 mmol/mol); lower HbA1c—6% (42 mmol/mol) is optimal if it can be achieved without significant hypoglycemia; also, the target may be relaxed to 7% (53 mmol/mol) in order to prevent hypoglycemia [7, 8].

2. Lifestyle intervention

After diagnosis GD, to reach the goals for plasma glucose levels, the first step is the initiation of a lifestyle intervention program (including medical nutrition therapy—MNT and physical activity—PA).

MNT is the cornerstone of the GDM treatment. MNT alone can assure glycemic targets in 80–90% of GDM patients [9]. Maternal height and weight are key factors for the medical nutrition therapy, providing adequate calories and nutrients for both maternal and fetal nutrition, maintaining glycemic targets and the absence of ketones with appropriate weight gain [10–12]. For a GDM mother with a normal body mass index (BMI) of 18.5–24.9 kg/m^2, the number of adequate calories is about 30 kcal/kg [9]. Nevertheless, since more than 60% of women diagnosed with GDM are overweight or obese, a caloric restriction is needed. The ADA states that no research identifies a specific optimal calorie intake for women with GDM and that the calorie needs are no different from those of pregnant women without GDM [7]. Therefore, ADA issued only general recommendations (following the dietary reference intakes) for 175 g of carbohydrate, 71 g of protein, 28 g of fiber, emphasizing the importance of the amount and type of carbohydrate with significant impact concerning the glucose levels, especially postprandial glucose peak [7]. ADA recommends individualized nutrition plan developed by a registered dietitian familiar with the management of GDM [7]. The National Institute for Health and Care Excellence (NICE) guidelines recommend a healthy diet, emphasizing the importance of low glycemic index foods (that should replace those with a high glycemic index) for GDM women; also there is the recommendation for a dietitian when GDM is present [13].

The carbohydrate intake should be reduced to 33–45% of the total calories, and distributed over 3 meals, and 2–4 snacks/day, thus reducing postprandial glucose peak [8, 14], while as the rest of the calories should be divided between protein (20%) and lipids (40%) [15].

Excessive weight gain during pregnancy should be avoided for GDM women [16]. The weight gain during pregnancy depends on pre-pregnancy BMI:

- 12.5–18 kg of weight gain for underweight women (BMI <18.5 kg/m^2);
- 11.5–16 kg for normal weight (BMI 18.5–24.9 kg/m^2);
- 7–11.5 kg for overweight (BMI 25–29.9 kg/m^2)
- 5–9 kg for obese (BMI ≥30.0 kg/m^2) [17]

Physical activity improves glycemic control in GDM women. The generally accepted recommendation is daily moderate-intensity regular exercise (walking 30 minutes/day or more—if no medical contraindications) improves blood glucose control [13, 14].

3. Pharmacological treatment

Pharmacological treatment is recommended when lifestyle intervention does not reduce hyperglycemia to reach the glycemic target. There is no international consensus on when to start pharmacological treatment of GDM [18]. The Canadian Diabetes Association (CDA) and NICE guidelines, both recommend beginning pharmacological treatment if glycemic control is not achieved after 1–2 weeks of lifestyle intervention [13, 19].

Oral antidiabetic medication has been described in a previous chapter. The authors want to resume the most important clinical implications and the comparisons with insulin treatment.

3.1 Metformin

The use of metformin in GDM after the glycemic target is not reached with lifestyle intervention is recommended by the NICE guidelines [13]. Metformin is classified as a category B drug, which implies that there is no evidence of animal, or fetal toxicity or teratogenicity. In general, metformin appears to be a safe alternative to insulin for the GDM treatment, but it crosses the placenta, and it may be present in a higher concentration in the fetal circulation than in the maternal circulation [19]. Studies were performed for the assessment of metformin exposure in-utero. There is no evidence that the metformin is affecting the fetus with regards to an early motor, linguistic, social, [20], metabolic [20, 21], and neurodevelopmental [22, 23] outcomes, but long-term follow up studies are needed. The metformin was associated with a lower risk of neonatal hypoglycemia and less maternal weight gain than insulin in two systematic reviews [24, 25]. Almost half of the patients with GDM who were initially treated with metformin needed insulin to achieve acceptable glucose control [26]. Metformin remains an option as a second line treatment in GDM women who refuse insulin treatment or who are unable to administer insulin safely.

3.2 Glyburide

Glyburide (glibenclamide) was associated with increased birth weight, macrosomia and neonatal hypoglycemia compared with insulin [20, 25], and similar to metformin, crosses the placenta [27]. Glyburide therapy during pregnancy is not recommended as first- or second-line treatment, but it may be used as third-line treatment if insulin is refused, and metformin is either refused or insufficient to reach targeted glycemic control [19].

There is no human data for the use of any other antihyperglycemic medication in the treatment of GDM (DPP-4 inhibitors, GLP-1 receptor agonists or SGLT2 inhibitors) [19]. Patients treated with oral therapy should be informed that they cross the placenta. No adverse effects on the fetus have been demonstrated; long-term studies are lacking [7].

3.3 Insulin therapy

Insulin is the first-line antihyperglycemic medication recommended for treatment of GDM [7, 19]. None of the currently available insulin preparations has been demonstrated to cross the placenta [7]. If glycemic control is not achieved after 1–2 weeks of lifestyle intervention, insulin treatment should be initiated [19]. Insulin remains the gold standard treatment for GDM women that do not reach glycemic targets with lifestyle intervention, as recommended by several guidelines (see **Table 1** below). Insulin use reduces fetal and maternal morbidity [28, 29].

International Federation of Gynecology and Obstetrics (FIGO), 2015	- Oral therapy failure or - One of the risk factors: • Diagnosing diabetes before 20 weeks of gestation • Oral therapy for more than 30 weeks • Fasting plasma blood glucose above 110 mg/dl • 1-hour postprandial glycemia above 140 mg/dl • Weight gain over 12 kilograms during pregnancy
Canadian Diabetes Association (CDA), 2018	If glycemic control is not achieved in 2 weeks after the initiation of medical, nutritional intervention
American Diabetes Association (ADA), 2018	First line therapy if glycemic control is not achieved after diet intervention
American College of Obstetricians and Gynecologists (ACOG), 2018	First line therapy if glycemic control is not achieved after diet intervention

Table 1.
Insulin initiation recommendations.

3.3.1 Types of insulin

3.3.1.1 Human insulin

3.3.1.1.1 Regular insulin

Regular insulin (U-100, U-500) is identical to human insulin, and it is used as meal-time insulin to cover postprandial hyperglycemia. Its time to onset is about 30 minutes (10–75 minutes), the peak effect is in 3 hours (2.5–5 hours), and the effect ends at about 8 hours (up to 24 hours for U500). The FDA pregnancy category is B [30].

3.3.1.1.2 Human insulin inhalation (nasal insulin)

Human insulin inhalation (nasal insulin) is equivalent unit-for-unit to insulin lispro. Its onset is 15 minutes, and its peak action time is ~50 minutes. Duration of action is about 2 hours. Inhaled human insulin carries a boxed warning for broncho-spasms in patients with chronic lung disease. It is a pregnancy category C drug [30].

3.3.1.2 Rapid-acting insulin analogs

Another analog of human insulin is insulin aspart produced from *Saccharomyces cerevisiae*, a type of yeast. Aspart should be taken 5–10 minutes before a meal. It can be used like for multiple subcutaneous injections or in insulin pumps. Its peak action time is 40–50 minutes, and its duration of action is 3–5 hours. Insulin aspart produce less hypoglycemia than the regular insulin [31]. The FDA pregnancy category is B and can be used in pregnancy. Data from two clinical trials (349 exposed pregnancies) do not indicate any adverse effect on pregnancy or fetal/neonatal health compared with human insulin [30].

3.3.1.2.1 Insulin aspart

Insulin aspart was introduced on the market with nicotinamide and L-arginine hydrochloride as excipients to enhance its absorption. Although the active molecule is identical, there are no available data for its use in pregnancy and its excretion in human milk [30].

3.3.1.2.2 Insulin lispro

Insulin lispro (U-100 and U-200) is an analog produced in *Escherichia coli* cultures. Its onset of action is 10–15 minutes. The peak is at 30–90 minutes, and its duration of action is 3–4 hours. Also, it can be used in insulin pumps or pens. The U-100 and U-200 formulations have the same bioequivalence and pharmacokinetics. The FDA pregnancy category is B and can be used in pregnancy. The data from a large number of exposed pregnancies do not indicate any adverse effect on pregnancy or fetal/neonatal health [30].

3.3.1.2.3 Insulin glulisine

Insulin glulisine is a recombinant insulin. It is obtained using *Escherichia coli*. It works fast nearly in 10–15 minutes. Its peak installs in 55 minutes, and its full duration is 4–5 hours. Although it can be used in some insulin pumps, it is not approved for all pump brands. The FDA pregnancy category is C. In this case, the vigilance should be given when prescribing glulisine to pregnant women, and the drug should only be used if the potential benefit justifies the potential risk to the fetus. There are limited data (less than 300 pregnancy outcomes) from the use of insulin glulisine in pregnant women [30].

3.3.1.3 Intermediate insulin

3.3.1.3.1 Insulin isophane

Insulin isophane (NPH) is an intermediate-acting insulin. It is also produced in *Escherichia coli*. It is similar to human insulin and is presented in a liquid suspension. Its onset of action is maximum 2 hours, with an average peak of 4 hours. NPH full duration of action is 10–20 hours. No restrictions on use in gestational diabetes or pregnancy; do not cross the placental barrier. The FDA pregnancy category is B [30].

3.3.1.4 Basal analogs

3.3.1.4.1 Insulin detemir

Insulin detemir (U-100) is a long-acting analog produced in *Saccharomyces cerevisiae*. Detemir insulin lacks a defined peak and lasts for up to 24 hours, and time to onset of action can be 1–2 hours. The detemir insulin has less incidence of hypoglycemia compared to NPH regimen in pregnant women [32]. The FDA pregnancy category is B; considered during pregnancy. The potential benefit must be considered against the possible increased risk of adverse pregnancy outcomes. One clinical trial suggests a possible increased risk of serious adverse maternal outcomes compared with isophane insulin and data from an additional 250 outcomes from pregnant women exposed to insulin detemir suggest no maternal or fetal/neonatal toxicity [30].

3.3.1.4.2 Insulin glargine

Insulin glargine (U-100) is a long-acting analog produced in *Escherichia coli*. The acidic solution is neutralized in subcutaneous tissue, and micro precipitates are formed. These micro precipitates slowly release glargine over 24 hours. Its onset of action is 1–2 hours, its duration of action are 24 hours and has no peak. The FDA pregnancy category was previously C, no human pregnancy data. May be considered during pregnancy, if necessary, but we do not have clinical data on exposed pregnancies from controlled clinical studies available. The data from pregnant women (between 300 and 1000 pregnancy outcomes) indicate no adverse effects on pregnancy, nor malformations or feto-neonatal toxicity [30].

3.3.1.4.3 Insulin glargine

Insulin glargine (U-300) is a long-acting insulin. It is not bioequivalent to glargine U-100, but it had the same structure and was approved in February 2015. Glargine U-300 is produced in *Escherichia coli*. Its peak action develops over 6 hours and continues for an entire 24 hours. The serum concentrations decline after 16–36 hours. It is dosed once daily. There is no clinical experience until now with the use of insulin glargine (U-300) in pregnant women [30].

3.3.1.4.4 Insulin degludec

Insulin degludec U-100 and U-200 are considered bioequivalent. The insulin degludec's mode of slow absorption and prolonged action is based on the formation of soluble multi-hexamers. Insulin degludec onset of action is nearly 1 hour and has no peak. It is dosed once daily. It can be dosed at any time of the day because of its long duration of action. There is no clinical experience in pregnant women [30].

3.3.2 Insulin regimens

There are many insulin regimens proposed for treating hyperglycemia, but the multiple daily injections (MDI) is by far the most efficient and the most flexible [33].

The insulin regimen should be chosen based on the blood glucose profile. Therefore, if fasting glycaemia is higher than 90–95 mg/dl, basal insulin should be initiated. It can be a long-acting insulin analog or neutral protamine Hagedorn. The basal insulin dose can be calculated according to the weight: 0.2 units/kg/day.

If the hyperglycemia follows a meal, than rapid-acting insulin or regular insulin should be initiated before that m74eal (begin with 1 u of insulin for 10–15 g of carbohydrates).

Sometimes both fasting and postprandial glycaemia are elevated, thereby needing MDI: 3 mealtime insulin and basal insulin. The total daily insulin requirement during the first trimester, is 0.7 units/kg/day, while in the second trimester it is 0.8 units/kg/day, and in the third trimester, it is 0.9–1.0 units/kg/day. This does not necessarily fit all pregnancies. Usually, in pregestational diabetes, the total insulin dose is up to twice higher than in GDM.

In the case of morbid obesity, the initial doses of insulin can be increased to 1.5–2.0 units/kg to overcome the combined IR of pregnancy and obesity [9].

Usually, the calculated total daily dose of insulin should be divided in two as for type 1 and type 2 diabetes: 50% as basal insulin at bedtime, and 50% divided between 3 meals and given as rapid-acting, or regular insulin before meals.

The doses of insulin have to be continuously optimized, so the self-monitoring blood glucose is essential.

Rapid-acting insulin analogs are preferred over regular insulin in pregnancy because there is a lower risk of hypoglycemia, and because they provide a better postprandial blood glucose control [29, 33].

3.3.3 Insulin initiation

Insulin initiation is synthesized in **Table 1**.

3.4 Glycemic targets and control

Blood glucose control in important in gestational diabetes because it confers the future mother a sense of disease control and validation that diet and treatment are doing their effect as the glycemic control improves, the risk of maternal and fetal complications decreases, a principle that was demonstrated by HAPO study results [34]. The results of this landmark study and other seven randomized trials have been included in a Cochrane analysis that compared the treatment of gestational diabetes mellitus (GDM) with standard care. It demonstrated a lower risk of a composite endpoint (death, shoulder dystocia, humerus, clavicle fracture or nerve palsy), and also a lower risk of pre-eclampsia and macrosomia (birth weight over 4000 g or 90th percentile), with no differences between oral and injectable treatment [35].

Thereby, gestational auto monitoring and surveillance by an obstetrician in collaboration with the diabetologist, nutritionist and midwife is essential for achieving glycemic targets during pregnancy, labor and after birth. These targets are synthesized in **Tables 2** and **3**.

3.5 Methods for glucose monitoring

3.5.1 Glycated hemoglobin (HbA1c)

Although glycated hemoglobin values must be interpreted with caution in patients with dilution anemia, iron deficiency anemia or other hematological

5th International Workshop Conference Gestational Diabetes and International Association of Diabetes and Pregnancy Study Group, 2007	Capillary pre-prandial glucose <95 mg/dl (5.3 mmol/l) Capillary 1 hour post-prandial glucose <140 mg/dl (7.8 mmol/l) Capillary 2 hour post-prandial glucose <120 mg/dl (6.7 mmol/l)
FIGO, 2015	Capillary pre-prandial glucose <95 mg/dl (5.3 mmol/l) Capillary 1 hour post-prandial glucose <140 mg/dl (7.8 mmol/l) Capillary 2 hour post-prandial glucose <120 mg/dl (6.7 mmol/l)
CDA, 2018	Capillary pre-prandial glucose <95 mg/dl (5.3 mmol/l) Capillary 1 hour post-prandial glucose <140 mg/dl (7.8 mmol/l) Capillary 2 hour post-prandial glucose <120 mg/dl (6.7 mmol/l)
ADA, 2018	Capillary pre-prandial glucose <95 mg/dl (5.3 mmol/l) Capillary 1 hour post-prandial glucose <140 mg/dl (7.8 mmol/l) Capillary 2 hour post-prandial glucose <120 mg/dl (6.7 mmol/l)

Table 2.
Glycemic targets during pregnancy.

FIGO, 2015	Capillary glucose 72–126 mg/dl (4–7 mmol/l)
ACOG, 2018	Capillary glucose 70–110 mg/dl (3.9–3.1 mmol/l)

Table 3.
Glycemic targets during labor.

pathologies like minor thalassemia [36, 37], it proves to be useful in checking the self-reported date by the pregnant, especially if she is treated with insulin.

Other parameters that could be used for short-term (2–3 weeks) evaluation of blood glucose control is glycated albumin. It is not influenced by iron deficiency, but the values are low in nephrotic syndrome or thyroid disorders that sometimes are present in pregnancy. This marker was studied in GDM, but the cutoff limits are not precisely known with consideration of some population differences [38]. Molecules like fructosamine or 1,5-anhydroglucitol have not proven their utility [39–41].

3.5.2 Self-monitoring of capillary blood glucose (SMBG)

The efficiency of capillary blood testing (8 determinations per day) in pregnant diabetes patients has been demonstrated since the 1980s [42]. Current guidelines [7, 8, 12, 18] mention in general terms the frequency and optimal period (fasting, 1 or 2 hours postprandial) when a test should be done without customizing for treatment, previous glycemic control.

In healthy adult pregnant women, 1-hour glycemia during a glucose challenge test was a better marker for insulin sensibility, being correlated with a fetal abdominal circumference in echography [43]. In Jovanovic and collab study [42], glycemia at 1 hour after food intake in the third trimester was the best predictor for birth weight. Combs et al. used the same 1-hour glycemia to establish the best threshold (130 mg/dl) for which the risk for macrosomia and small for gestational age (SGA) is reduced [44]. Metzger was the one that proposed that 2-hours postprandial glycemia should be used in GDM with the limit of 120 mg/dl [34]. Two clinical studies compared the blood glucose determination concluding that 1-hour glycemia is superior, but with two important biases—lack of randomization and low statistical power [45, 46].

A randomized clinical trial demonstrated that patients who adjusted insulin doses based on 1-hour postprandial glycemia had a lower risk of giving birth to a macrosomia, or to have a cesarean procedure; also, the risk for neonatal hypoglycemia was smaller [47]. Not only the glycemic values *per se* is important, but also the pregnant women with GDM should be taught to estimate their carbohydrate intake and physical activity and adjust the insulin doses. Other factors that cannot be influenced are a hormonal secretion from the placenta, daily cortisol secretion variability that contributes to glucose excursions. Sivan et al. observed in their study a pattern in which 1-hour postprandial glycemia is abnormally raised in the morning, and 2 hours postprandial glycemia is abnormally raised in the evening [48].

The frequency of determination is as much as necessary. Based on a randomized control trial (RCT) the initial recommendation for SMBG is 4 tests per day, with the possibility to lessen the number of determinations according to if the patient has good control and the fetal morphology is normal [49]. In basal-bolus insulin-treated GDM 7 tests per day are recommended, but patient adherence is weak (a mean of 4.2 in an observational study) [50].

The limit for SMBG consists in the accuracy bias: lowering hematocrit by dilution makes the capillary glucose to be overestimated. Some glucometers have included in their software functions to correct the hematocrit values, but the majority uses colorimetric and amperometric methods that depend on it. Considering the tight glycemic control required during pregnancy and the fact that insulin doses are adjusted based on SMBG, some researchers recommend that the bias and imprecision should be set at below 2% and the meters be verified according to international quality criteria [51].

3.5.3 Continuous interstitial glucose monitoring (glucose sensors, CGMS)

Systems for interstitial glucose monitoring have been used together with insulin pumps in type 1 diabetes pregnancies in RCTs and observational studies [52, 53]. In GDM pregnancies data come from small observational studies where they showed benefit for disclosing high and low glycemic excursions missed by SMBG [54].

Glycemic sensors can be used as a guide for therapy initiation, as demonstrated by Kestilä et al. [55]. The anti-diabetes medication was introduced in a higher proportion of GDM women with CGMS versus SMBG. Nevertheless, there were not any significant differences for the perinatal endpoints. The long-term impact of glycemic control during pregnancy is not known; therefore, the benefit of this intervention must be balanced with unnecessary treatment. The techniques for monitoring blood glucose are summarized in **Table 4**.

All these efforts in using the best method for monitoring insulin therapy in GDM are to maintain glycemic control for preventing fetal and maternal complications.

3.6 Fetal complications associated with insulin therapy

3.6.1 Neonatal hypoglycemia

Glucose is a nutrient that freely crosses the placenta from maternal to fetal circulation, to assure the energy required for growth. Immediately after birth, the glucose source disappears with a physiologic "hypoglycemia" in the blood of the newborn that triggers the secretion of counterregulatory hormones (glucagon, steroids, catecholamines, growth hormone). In GDM pregnancies, the glycemia is continuously raised and determines a consecutive higher secretion of insulin that makes hypoglycemia more severe and prolonged than in normal newborns [56–59].

Regimen	SBGM	CGMS
GDM with diet or oral antidiabetics	Fasting 1 hour postprandial	- Fine-tune insulin dosing - Nocturnal hypoglycemia - Nocturnal hyperglycemia - Postprandial hyperglycemia
GDM with basal insulin	Fasting	
	1 hour postprandial	
	Bedtime	
GDM with premixed insulin	Fasting	
	1 hour postprandial	
	Dinner preprandial	
	1 hour postprandial	
GDM with basal bolus	Fasting	
	Preprandial (lunch, dinner)	
	1 hour postprandial	

Table 4.
Insulin glucose monitoring techniques [adapted from American Association of Clinical Endocrinologist and American College of Endocrinology].

Neonatal transient hypoglycemia could have implications in the neurocognitive development as was shown by magnetic resonance imaging [60]. Also, it has psychological implications on the mother-child relationship because they are separated after birth for treatment. Hence, based on their study results, Voormolen et al. recommend screening all newborns from GDM women in the first 12 hours after birth because the majority of the events occur in this interval, with a higher incidence being in the insulin-treated group [58].

A series of studies demonstrated that newborns of GDM patients that were treated with metformin had fewer hypoglycemic events than those of women treated with insulin [21, 61]. Insulin analogs have a lower rise in postprandial glycemic values without elevating hypoglycemic risk and should be preferred to human insulins [29, 33].

Regarding sulfonylureas, a meta-analysis demonstrated that glyburide treatment GDM had a higher risk of neonatal hypoglycemia and also macrosomia that the metformin-treated GDM [62].

3.6.2 Congenital anomalies

The relationship between insulin therapy and congenital anomalies was studied, especially in type 1 diabetes. The most important confounding factor is glycemic control. Although some case reports indicate an association between the use of insulin lispro and the risk of teratogenesis [63], another meta-analysis supports the fact that it is safe for use [64]. This risk could be explained by mitogenesis stimulation by binding with a higher affinity for IGF-1 receptors. Lispro insulin has a 1.5 and insulin glargine a 6.5 fold increase of receptor binding [65]. There are only retrospective studies that indicate glargine as safe insulin in pregnancy [66].

3.7 Birth complications associated with insulin therapy

3.7.1 Cesarean section (CS)

A Cochrane analysis of 1481 women with GDM showed that in the treatment group there was a higher number of induced labors versus the group with standard antenatal care, but with no difference regarding the number of births by CS [35]. Another meta-analysis did not demonstrate a correlation between the use of different types of insulin-like aspart, lispro and the birth by CS [67, 68]. Although the risk is not influenced by insulin treatment, it can be reduced by induction of labor (IOL) in 38th–39th week of gestation with better outcomes for the fetus [69].

3.7.2 Vacuum-assisted birth

Although pre-gestational diabetes raises the risk for vacuum assisted birth (shoulder dystocia, humerus, clavicle, skull fracture, Erb's palsy, subarachnoidian or subdural hemorrhages, asphyxia, convulsion), in GDM the risk was similar to that in the general population and could not be related to insulin therapy [68, 70]. A particular situation is with GDM that appeared in pregnancies obtained by assisted reproductive technology where the risk for perinatal and obstetrical complications is probably increased by the adverse effect of hyperglycemia, not by insulin treatment [71].

3.7.3 Fetal morbidity

Evidence that indicates a higher risk for fetal morbidity and mortality in GDM a scarce and less pronounced as in pre-gestational diabetes. Current decisions of IOL as compared to expectant management should be individualized because the studies lack in this area. An RCT that showed that there is no difference between the two strategies regarding morbidity, but the IOL reduces the risk for shoulder dystocia in the macrosomic fetus [72]. The use of insulin analogs like detemir does not influence the morbidity [73].

3.8 Maternal complications associated with insulin therapy

3.8.1 Maternal hypoglycemia

Hypoglycemia threshold is specific for every individual. In pregnancy, there is a reduction of this threshold by 20% [74]. Patients with GDM that are treated with insulin must maintain a glycemia above 3.7 mmol/l (66 mg/dl) according to CDA, or above 3.9 mmol/l (70 mg/dl) according to ADA [7].

Insulin analogs are superior to human insulin because the hypoglycemic events are less frequent in type 1 diabetic pregnancies [75]. The use of multiple daily injections is as effective as continuous subcutaneous insulin infusion [76].

Maternal hypoglycemia affects the fetus just in severe cases when is associated with loss of consciousness or secondary to trauma. Also, it was observed that repeated episodes could lead to growth over the 90th percentile [77]. These episodes are more likely to be present in the first trimester in women who had pregestational diabetes than in GDM [74].

3.8.2 Hypertension

There is moderate quality evidence that indicates higher hypertension associated hypertension without giving details in insulin-treated GDM. This fact should be further researched because it is in contradiction with a non-modified risk for pre-eclampsia [68].

3.9 Intrapartum management

During the latent phase of labor hepatic gluconeogenesis is sufficient for providing the caloric requirements, but becomes exiguous during the active phase when intravenous glucose is perfused.

The study of Rosenberg and collab. demonstrated there is no significant difference in neonatal hypoglycemia, neonatal injury, Apgar score at 1–5 minutes in patients with insulin therapy that were managed with two approaches: dextrose 5% 125 ml/h with a simultaneous insulin drip (adjustable rate 0.5–2.5 u/h) or dextrose 5% alternating with ringer lactate (125 ml/h) and insulin introduction when the targets are exceeded [77]. Other researchers recommend dextrose 10% with an insulin drip [78].

Lowering maternal glycemia is necessary for preventing neonatal hypoglycemia, balancing this risk with that for ketosis. Capillary blood glucose should be tested every hour and urinary ketone bodies every time is possible [77]. ACOG agreed to the protocol proposed by Coustan [79] for maintaining a mean intrapartum glycemic value of 100 mg/dl. For this, blood glucose should be tested every 2 hours with adjustments in insulin perfusion rates.

Women with GDM or type 2 diabetes, which were treated with oral therapy have a low insulin requirement and in most cases do not need treatment during labor. Thus, CDA recommends a “watchful waiting” and insulin initiation just in cases where glycemia is above 146 mg/dl (7.0 mmol/l) [19]. Ryan mentions the same principle in a review published before—if GDM pregnant had a necessary below 0.5 u/kg/day, they could be initially monitored. Otherwise, patients with type 1 diabetes or type 2, GDM with a necessary above this limit will need insulin perfusions [78]. Insulin perfusion rates could be adjusted using sliding scales as proposed by Dude [80].

Although most of the studies use protocols for intravenous insulin administration, patients with insulin pumps can choose to keep their device during labor [81, 82]. This is recommended in centers with experience because during labor they can become unable to handle the pump given the pain, or some incidents like catheter avulsion could appear. In these cases, the patient is informed that a switch to an insulin drip is needed [19].

Another problem comes out when betamethasone is administered for premature birth. In patients with type 1 diabetes, an increase up to 40% of all doses during the next 5 days assures an adequate glycemic control [83]. A retrospective analysis of insulin drips in pregnant with GDM injected by a standard anticipatory protocol and with higher doses was associated with improving glycemic variability and decreasing by 25% the absolute risk for neonatal hypoglycemia [84].

3.10 Postpartum management

Insulin requirements drop quickly after giving birth and women are exposed to hypoglycemia. Patients with GDM usually do not need insulin, and women with type 1 and type 2 diabetes return to the previous regimen, but at doses that are at 60% of the antepartum necessary [85]. In the case where the doses are not remembered, half of the third-trimester dose could be injected. Another alternative is calculating dose per kilogram. With an insulin pump, the doctor will titrate downward the basal rate and boluses on a similar algorithm or adjust based on the information from glucose sensors for newer models.

Breastfeeding influences insulin sensibility: as the frequency of lactation increases, the HOMA and ISI (0, 120) have better values [86], so during breastfeeding the insulin requirement falls by 10% [87].

3.11 Future research directions

There is a lot of missing evidence in optimal treatment for GDM. Insulin treatment could be improved by developing automatic algorithms for calculating the appropriate doses like that proposed by Dinglas [88]. Moreover, fetal morbidity can be influenced by better monitoring like using glucose sensors that are more accurate in the hypoglycemic range [89–91].

Micro-RNAs are now extensively studied in different domains and might apply to diagnosing and selecting GDM patients that require insulin treatment [92].

Not eventually, the whole perspective of insulin therapy will change if the oral bioavailability of this peptide hormone will be enhanced. Polymeric nanocarriers and mucoadhesive discs were studied in diabetic rats and are the future expectation for mothers with diabetes [93].

Acknowledgements

All authors had an equal contribution and shared the first authorship.

Conflict of interest

None.

Notes/thanks/other declarations

This chapter was financed by Novo Nordisk.

Author details

Anca Pantea-Stoian*, Roxana Adriana Stoica and Simona Diana Stefan
Nutrition and Metabolic Diseases Department, "Carol Davila" University of Medicine and Pharmacy Diabetes, Bucharest, Romania

*Address all correspondence to: ancastoian@yahoo.com

References

[1] World Health Organisation and Department of Non-Communicable Disease Surveillance. Definition, Diagnosis and Classification of Diabetes Mellitus and its Complications. Part 1. Geneva: WHO; 1999

[2] International Association of Diabetes and Pregnancy Study Groups Consensus Panel, Metzger BE, Gabbe SG, Persson B, Buchanan TA, Catalano PA, et al. International association of diabetes and pregnancy study groups recommendations on the diagnosis and classification of hyperglycemia in pregnancy. Diabetes Care. 2010;**33**: 676-682. PMID: 20190296

[3] Caprio S. Development of type 2 diabetes mellitus in the obese adolescent: A growing challenge. Endocrine Practice. 2012;**18**:791-795

[4] Ferrara A. Increasing prevalence of gestational diabetes mellitus: A public health perspective. Diabetes Care. 2007;**30**(Suppl 2):S141-S146

[5] American College of Obstetricians and Gynecologists. ACOG practice bulletin: Assessment of risk factors for preterm birth: Clinical management guidelines for obstetrician-gynecologists: Number 31. Obstetrics and Gynecology. 2001;**98**:709-716

[6] Metzger BE, Buchanan TA, Coustan DR, de Leiva A, Dunger DB, Hadden DR, et al. Summary and recommendations of the fifth international workshop-conference on gestational diabetes mellitus. Diabetes Care. 2007;**30**(Suppl 2):S251-S260. DOI: 10.2337/dc07-s225

[7] American Diabetes Association. Management of diabetes in pregnancy: Standards of medical care in diabetes. Diabetes Care. 2018;**41**(Suppl.1):S137-S143. DOI: 10.2337/dc18-S013

[8] American College of Obstetricians and Gynecologists. Committee on practice bulletins—Obstetrics. ACOG practice bulletin No. 190: Gestational diabetes mellitus. Obstetrics and Gynecology. 2018;**131**(2):e49-e64. DOI: 10.1097/AOG.0000000000002501

[9] Jovanovic L. Role of diet and insulin treatment of diabetes in pregnancy. Clinical Obstetrics and Gynecology. 2000;**43**:46-55

[10] Beaser RS et al. Joslin's Diabetes Deskbook, A Guide for Primary Care Providers. 2nd ed. Lippincott: Wiliams & Wilkins; 2010. pp. 595-601

[11] American Diabetes Association, Bantle JP, Wylie-Rosett J, Albright AL, Apovian CM, Clark NG, et al. Nutrition recommendations and interventions for diabetes: A position statement of the American Diabetes Association. Diabetes Care. 2008;**31**:S61-S78

[12] The International Federation of Gynecology and Obstetrics (FIGO) Initiative on gestational diabetes mellitus: A pragmatic guide for diagnosis, management, and care. International Journal of Gynecology & Obstetrics. 2015;**13**(1):S173-S211. DOI: 10.1016/S0020-7292(15)30007-2

[13] Diabetes in Pregnancy: Management from Preconception to the Postnatal Period NICE Guideline. 2015. Available from: www.nice.org.uk/guidance/ng3

[14] Blumer I, Hadar E, Hadden DR, Jovanovič L, Mestman JH, Murad MH, et al. Diabetes and pregnancy: An endocrine society clinical practice guideline. The Journal of Clinical Endocrinology and Metabolism. 2013;**98**:4227-4249

[15] Mulford MI, Jovanovic-Peterson L, Peterson CM. Alternative therapies for the management of gestational diabetes. Clinics in Perinatology. 1993;**20**:619-634

[16] Cheng YW, Chung JH, Kurbisch-Block I, Inturrisi M, Shafer S, Caughey AB. Gestational weight gain and gestational diabetes mellitus: Perinatal outcomes. Obstetrics and Gynecology. 2008;**112**:1015-1022

[17] Rasmussen KM, Catalano PM, Yaktine AL. New guidelines for weight gain during pregnancy: What obstetrician/gynecologists should know. Current Opinion in Obstetrics & Gynecology. 2009;**21**:521-526

[18] Diagnostic Criteria and Classification of Hyperglycaemia First Detected in Pregnancy. World Health Organization; 2013. PMID: 24199271

[19] Diabetes Canada Clinical Practice Guidelines Expert Committee. Diabetes Canada: Clinical practice guidelines for the prevention and management of diabetes in Canada. Canadian Journal of Diabetes. 2018;**42**(Suppl 1):S1-S325

[20] Ijäs H, Vääräsmäki M, Saarela T, et al. A follow-up of a randomised study of metformin and insulin in gestational diabetes mellitus: Growth and development of the children at the age of 18 months. BJOG. 2015;**122**:994-1000

[21] Rowan JA, Rush EC, Obolonkin V, et al. Metformin in gestational diabetes: The offspring follow-up (MiG TOFU): Body composition at 2 years of age. Diabetes Care. 2011;**34**:2279-2284

[22] Tertti K, Eskola E, Ronnemaa T, et al. Neurodevelopment of two-year-old children exposed to metformin and insulin in gestational diabetes mellitus. Journal of Developmental and Behavioral Pediatrics. 2015;**36**:752-757

[23] Wouldes TA, Battin M, Coat S, et al. Neurodevelopmental outcome at 2 years in offspring of women randomised to metformin or insulin treatment for gestational diabetes. Archives of Disease in Childhood. Fetal and Neonatal Edition. 2016;**101**:F488-F493

[24] Balsells M, García-Patterson A, Sola I, Roqué M, Gich I, Corcoy R. Glibenclamide, metformin, and insulin for the treatment of gestational diabetes: A systematic review and meta-analysis. BMJ. 2015;**350**:h102

[25] Jiang Y-F, Chen X-Y, Ding T, Wang X-F, Zhu Z-N, Su S-W. Comparative efficacy and safety of OADs in management of GDM: Network meta-analysis of randomized controlled trials. The Journal of Clinical Endocrinology and Metabolism. 2015;**100**:2071-2080

[26] Rowan JA, Hague WM, Gao W, Battin MR, Moore MP, MiG Trial Investigators. Metformin versus insulin for the treatment of gestational diabetes. The New England Journal of Medicine. 2008;**358**:2003-2015

[27] Hebert MF, Ma X, Naraharisetti SB, et al. Obstetric-fetal pharmacology research unit network. Are we optimizing gestational diabetes treatment with glyburide? The pharmacologic basis for better clinical practice. Clinical Pharmacology and Therapeutics. 2009;**85**:607-614

[28] Hadden DR. When and how to start insulin treatment in gestational diabetes: A UK perspective. Diabetic Medicine. 2001;**18**:960-964

[29] Mecacci F, Carignani L, Cioni R, et al. Maternal metabolic control and perinatal outcome in women with gestational diabetes treated with regular or lispro insulin: Comparison with non-diabetic pregnant women. European Journal of Obstetrics, Gynecology, and Reproductive Biology. 2003;**111**:19-24

[30] European Medicines Agency. European Medicines Agency. Available from: http://www.ema.europa.eu/ema/ [Accessed: November 2, 2018]

[31] Mathiesen ER, Kinsley B, Amiel SA, et al. Maternal glycemic control and hypoglycemia in type 1 diabetic

pregnancy: A randomized trial of insulin aspart versus human insulin in 322 pregnant women. Diabetes Care. 2007;**30**:771-776

[32] Herrera KM, Rosenn BM, Foroutan J, et al. Randomized controlled trial of insulin detemir versus NPH for the treatment of pregnant women with diabetes. American Journal of Obstetrics and Gynecology. 2015;**213**:426.e1-426.e7

[33] Pettitt DJ, Ospina P, Kolaczynski JW, et al. Comparison of an insulin analog, insulin aspart, and regular human insulin with no insulin in gestational diabetes mellitus. Diabetes Care. 2003;**26**:183-186

[34] HAPO Study Cooperative Research Group, Metzger BE, Lowe LP, Dyer AR, Trimble ER, Chaovarindr U, et al. Hyperglycemia and adverse pregnancy outcomes. The New England Journal of Medicine. 2008;**358**:1991-2002. DOI: 10.1056/NEJMoa0707943

[35] Alwan N, Tuffnell DJ, West J. Treatments for gestational diabetes. Cochrane Database of Systematic Reviews. 2009;**8**(3):CD003395. DOI: 10.1002/14651858.CD003395.pub2

[36] Zhang X, Xiao Y, Fan Y. Investigating the reliability of HbA1c monitoring for blood glucose control during late pregnancy in patients with gestational diabetes mellitus (GDM) with and without β-thalassemia minor. Diabetes Therapy. 2018;**9**(6):2305-2313. DOI: 10.1007/s13300-018-0516-z

[37] Koga M, Morita S, Saito H, Mukai M, Kasayama S. Association of erythrocyte indices with glycated haemoglobin in pre-menopausal women. Diabetic Medicine: A Journal of The British Diabetic Association. 2007;**24**:843-847

[38] Shimizu I, Hiramatsu Y, Omori Y, Nakabayashi M. Glycated albumin reflects maternal and perinatal outcome in a multicenter study of Japan. Diabetes Pregnancy. 2010;**10**:27-31 (in Japanese) Abstract

[39] Delgado MR, Novik AV, Cardemil MF, Santander AD. Plasma fructosamine to evaluate metabolic control among women with gestational diabetes. Revista Médica de Chile. 2011;**139**:1444-1450

[40] Tetsuo M, Hamada T, Yoshimatsu K, Ishimatsu J, Matsunaga T. Serum levels of 1,5-anhydro-d-glucitol during the normal and diabetic pregnancy and puerperium. Acta Obstetricia et Gynecologica Scandinavica. 1990;**69**:479-485

[41] Mendes N, Tavares Ribeiro R, Serrano F. Beyond self-monitored plasma glucose and HbA1c: The role of non-traditional glycaemic markers in gestational diabetes mellitus. Journal of Obstetrics and Gynaecology. 2018 Aug;**38**(6):762-769. DOI: 10.1080/01443615.2017.1412409

[42] Jovanovic L, Peterson CM, Saxena BB, Dawood MY, Saudek CD. Feasibility of maintaining normal glucose profiles in insulin-dependent pregnant diabetic women. The American Journal of Medicine. 1980;**68**:105-112

[43] Parretti E, Mecacci F, Papini M, et al. Third-trimester maternal glucose levels from diurnal profiles in nondiabetic pregnancies. Diabetes Care. 2001;**24**:1319-1323. PMID: 11473063

[44] Combs CA, Gunderson E, Kitzmiller JL, et al. Relationship of fetal macrosomia to maternal postprandial glucose control during pregnancy. Diabetes Care. 1992;**15**:1251-1257

[45] Moses RG, Lucas EM, Knights S. Gestational diabetes mellitus, At what time should the postprandial glucose level be monitored? Australian and New Zealand Journal of Obstetrics and Gynaecology. 1999;**39**(4):457-460. PMID: 10687763

[46] Weisz B, Shrim A, Homko CJ, et al. One hour versus two-hour postprandial glucose mesurement in gestational diabetes—A prospective study. Journal of Perinatology. 2005;**25**(4):241-244. DOI: 10.1038/sj.jp.7211243

[47] de Veciana M, Major CA, Morgan MA, et al. Postprandial versus preprandial blood glucose monitoring in women with gestational diabetes mellitus requiring insulin therapy. The New England Journal of Medicine. 1995;**333**(19):1237-1241. DOI: 10.1056/NEJM199511093331901

[48] Sivan E, Weisz B, Homko C, et al. One or two hours postprandial glucose measurements: Are they the same? American Journal of Obstetrics and Gynecology. 2001;**185**:604-607. DOI: 10.1067/mob.2001.117184

[49] Crowther CA, Hiller JE, Moss JR, et al. Effect of treatment of gestational diabetes mellitus on pregnancy outcomes. The New England Journal of Medicine. 2005;**352**(24):2477-2486. DOI: 10.1056/NEJMoa042973

[50] Langer O, Levy J, Brustaman L, et al. Glycemic control in gestational diabetes mellitus-how tight is tight enough: Small for gestational age versus large for gestational age? American Journal of Obstetrics and Gynecology. 1989;**161**(3):646-653. PMID: 2782347

[51] Immanuel J, Simmons D. A perspective on the accuracy of blood glucose meters during pregnancy. Diabetes Care. 2018;**41**(10):2053-2058. DOI: 10.2337/dc18-0833

[52] Rys PM, Ludwig-Slomczynska AH, Cyganek K, Malecki MT. Continuous subcutaneous insulin infusion vs multiple daily injections in pregnant women with type 1 diabetes mellitus: A systematic review and meta-analysis of randomised controlled trials and observational studies. European Journal of Endocrinology. 2018;**178**(5):545-563. DOI: 10.1530/EJE-17-0804

[53] Feig DS, Corcoy R, Donovan LE, et al. Pumps or multiple daily injections in pregnancy involving type 1 diabetes: A prespecified analysis of the CONCEPTT randomized trial. Diabetes Care. 2018;**41**(12):2471-2479. DOI: 10.2337/dc18-1437

[54] Chen R, Yogev Y, Ben-Haroush A, Jovanovic L, Hod M, Phillip M. Continuous glucose monitoring for the evaluation and improved control of gestational diabetes mellitus. The Journal of Maternal-Fetal & Neonatal Medicine. 2003;**14**:256-260

[55] Kestilä KK, Ekblad UU, Rönnemaa T. Continuous glucose monitoring versus self-monitoring of blood glucose in the treatment of gestational diabetes mellitus. Diabetes Research and Clinical Practice. 2007;**77**(2):174-179

[56] Rowan JA, Gao W, Hague WM, McIntyre HD. Glycemia and its relationship to outcomes in the metformin in gestational diabetes trial. Diabetes Care. 2010;**33**:9-16. DOI: 10.2337/ dc09-1407

[57] Nicholson W, Bolen S, Witkop CT, Neale D, Wilson L, Bass E. Benefits and risks of oral diabetes agents compared with insulin in women with gestational diabetes: A systematic review. Obstetrics and Gynecology. 2009;**113**:193-205. DOI: 10.1097/AOG.0b013e318190a459

[58] Voormolen DN, de Wit L, van Rijn BP, et al. Neonatal hypoglycemia following diet-controlled and insulin-treated gestational diabetes mellitus. Diabetes Care. 2018:1-7. DOI: 10.2337/dc18-0048

[59] Hawdon JM. Definition of neonatal hypoglycemia: Time for a rethink? Archives of Disease in Childhood. Fetal and Neonatal Edition. 2013;**98**:F382-F383. DOI: 10.1136/archdischild-2012-303422

[60] McKinlay CJD, Alsweiler JM, Ansell JM, et al. Neonatal hypoglycemia and neurodevelopmental outcomes at 2 years. The New England Journal of Medicine. 2015;**373**:1507-1518. DOI: 10.1056/NEJMoa1504909

[61] Simeonova-Krstevska S, Bogoev M, et al. Maternal and neonatal outcomes in pregnant women with gestational diabetes mellitus treated with diet, metformin or insulin. Open Access Macedonian Journal of Medical Sciences. 2018;**6**(5):803-807. DOI: 10.3889/oamjms.2018.200

[62] Zeng YC, Li MJ, Chen Y, Jiang L, Wang SM, Mo XL, et al. The use of glyburide in the management of gestational diabetes mellitus: A meta-analysis. Advances in Medical Sciences. 2014;**59**:95-101. DOI: 10.1016/j.advms.2014.03.001

[63] Diamond T, Kormas N. Possible adverse fetal effect of insulin lispro. The New England Journal of Medicine. 1997;**337**(14):1009-1010

[64] Nørgaard K, Sukumar N, Rafnsson SB, Saravanan P. Efficacy and safety of rapid-acting insulin analogs in special populations with type 1 diabetes or gestational diabetes: Systematic review and meta-analysis. Diabetes Therapy. 2018;**9**(3):891-917. DOI: 10.1007/s13300-018-0411-7

[65] Kurtzhals P, Schaffer L, Sorensen A, et al. Correlations of receptor binding and metabolic and mitogenic potencies of insulin analogs designed for clinical use. Diabetes. 2000;**49**:999-1005

[66] Callesen NF, Damm J, Mathiesen JM, et al. Treatment with the long-acting insulin analogues detemir or glargine during pregnancy in women with type 1 diabetes: Comparison of glycaemic control and pregnancy outcome. Journal of Maternal-Fetal and Neonatal Medicine. 2013;**26**:588-592

[67] Martis R, Crowther CA, Shepherd E, Alsweiler J, Downie MR, Brown J. Treatments for women with gestational diabetes mellitus: An overview of Cochrane systematic reviews. Cochrane Database of Systematic Reviews. 2018;**14**(8):CD012327. DOI: 10.1002/14651858.CD012327.pub2

[68] Brown J, Grzeskowiak L, Williamson K, Downie MR, Crowther CA. Insulin for the treatment of women with gestational diabetes. Cochrane Database of Systematic Reviews. 2017;**5**(11):CD012037. DOI: 10.1002/14651858.CD012037.pub2

[69] Melamed N, Ray JG, Geary M, et al. Induction of labor before 40 weeks is associated with lower rate of cesarean delivery in women with gestational diabetes mellitus. American Journal of Obstetrics and Gynecology. 2016;**214**(364):e1-e8

[70] Vitner D, Hiersch L, Ashwal E, Nassie D, Yogev Y, Aviram A. Outcomes of vacuum-assisted vaginal deliveries of mothers with gestational diabetes mellitus. The Journal of Maternal-Fetal & Neonatal Medicine. 2018;**2**:1-5. DOI: 10.1080/14767058.2018.1468880

[71] Kouhkan A, Khamseh ME, Pirjani R, et al. Obstetric and perinatal outcomes of singleton pregnancies conceived via assisted reproductive technology complicated by gestational diabetes mellitus: A prospective cohort study. BMC Pregnancy and Childbirth. 2018;**18**(1):495. DOI: 10.1186/s12884-018-2115-4

[72] Hod M, Mathiesen ER, Jovanovic L, et al. Perinatal outcomes in a randomized trial comparing insulin detemir with NPH in pregnant women with type 1 diabetes. The Journal of Maternal-Fetal & Neonatal Medicine. 2014;**27**(1):7-13. DOI: 10.3109/14767058.2013.799650

[73] Seaquist ER, Anderson J, Childs B, et al. Hypoglycemia and diabetes: A report of a workgroup of the American Diabetes Association and the Endocrine Society. Diabetes Care. 2013;**36**:1384-1395

[74] Toledano Y, Hadar E, Hod M. Safety of insulin analogues as compared with human insulin in pregnancy. Expert Opinion on Drug Safety. 2016;**15**(7):963-973. DOI: 10.1080/14740338.2016.1182153

[75] Farrar D, Tuffnell DJ, West J, West HM. Continuous subcutaneous insulin infusion versus multiple daily injections of insulin for pregnant women with diabetes. Cochrane Database of Systematic Reviews. 2016;**6**:CD005542

[76] Seaquist ER, Anderson J, Childs B, et al. Hypoglycemia and diabetes: A report of a workgroup of the American Diabetes Association and the Endocrine Society. Diabetes Care 2013;**36**:1384-95

[77] Rosenberg VA, Eglinton GS, Rauch ER, Skupski DW. Intrapartum maternal glycemic control in women with insulin requiring diabetes: A randomized clinical trial of rotating fluids versus insulin drip. American Journal of Obstetrics and Gynecology. 2006;**195**:1095-1099

[78] Ryan EA, Al-Agha R. Glucose control during labor and delivery. Current Diabetes Reports. 2014;**14**(1):450. DOI: 10.1007/s11892-013-0450-4

[79] Coustan DR, Carpenter MW. The diagnosis of gestational diabetes. Diabetes Care. 1998;**21**(Suppl 2):B5-B8. PMID: 9704220

[80] Dude A, Niznik CM, Szmuilowicz ED, Peaceman AM, Yee LM. Management of diabetes in the intrapartum and postpartum patient. American Journal of Perinatology. 2018;**35**(11):1119-1126. DOI: 10.1055/s-0038-1629903

[81] Drever E, Tomlinson G, Bai AD, et al. Insulin pump use compared with intra-venous insulin during labour and delivery: The INSPIRED observational cohort study. Diabetic Medicine. 2016;**33**:1253-1259

[82] Fresa R, Visalli N, Di Blasi V, et al. Experiences of continuous subcutaneous insulin infusion in pregnant women with type 1 diabetes during delivery from four Italian centers: A retrospective observational study. Diabetes Technology & Therapeutics. 2013;**15**:328-334

[83] Mathiesen ER, Christensen AB, Hellmuth E, Hornnes P, Stage E, Damm P. Insulin dose during glucocorticoid treatment for fetal lung maturation in diabetic pregnancy: Test of an algorithm [correction of analgoritm]. Acta Obstetricia et Gynecologica Scandinavica. 2002;**81**(9):835-839

[84] Rowe CW, Putt E, Brentnall O, Gebuehr A, Allabyrne J, Woods A, et al. An intravenous insulin protocol designed for pregnancy reduces neonatal hypoglycaemia following betamethasone administration in women with gestational diabetes. Diabetic Medicine. 2018. DOI: 10.1111/dme.13864

[85] Ringholm L, Mathiesen ER, Kelstrup L, Damm P. Managing type 1 diabetes mellitus in pregnancy-from planning to breastfeeding. Nature Reviews. Endocrinology. 2012;**8**(11):659-667. DOI: 10.1038/nrendo.2012.154

[86] Gunderson EP, Hedderson MM, Chiang V, Crites Y, Walton D, Azevedo RA, et al. Lactation intensity and postpartum maternal glucose tolerance and insulin resistance in women with recent GDM: The SWIFT cohort. Diabetes Care. 2012;**35**:50-56

[87] Riviello C, Mello G, Jovanovic LG. Breastfeeding and the basal insulin requirement in type 1 diabetic women. Endocrine Practice. 2009;**15**:187-193

[88] Dinglas C, Muscat J, Adams T, Peragallo-Dittko V, Vintzileos A, Heo HJ. Software-guided insulin dosing improves intrapartum glycemic management in women with diabetes mellitus. American Journal of Obstetrics and Gynecology. 2018;**219**(2):191.e1-191.e6. DOI: 10.1016/j.ajog.2018.05.003

[89] Harris DL, Bartin MR, Weston PJ, Harding JE. Continuous glucose monitoring in newborn babies at risk of hypoglycemia. The Journal of Pediatrics. 2010;**157**:198-202.e1

[90] Perri A, Giordano L, Corsello M, et al. Continuous glucose monitoring (CGM) in very low birth weight newborns needing parenteral nutrition: Validation and glycemic percentiles. Italian Journal of Pediatrics. 2018;**44**(1):99. DOI: 10.1186/s13052-018-0542-5

[91] McKinlay CJD, Chase JG, Dickson J, et al. Continuous glucose monitoring in neonates: A review. Maternal Health, Neonatology and Perinatology. 2017;**3**:18. DOI: 10.1186/s40748-017-0055-z

[92] Ibarra A, Vega-Guedes B, Brito-Casillas Y, Wägner AM. Diabetes in pregnancy and microRNAs: Promises and limitations in their clinical application. Non-Coding RNA. 2018;**4**(4):pii: E32. DOI: 10.3390/ncrna4040032

[93] Gedawy A, Martinez J, Al-Salami H, Dass CR. Oral insulin delivery: Existing barriers and current counter-strategies. The Journal of Pharmacy and Pharmacology. 2018;**70**(2):197-213. DOI: 10.1111/jphp.12852

Chapter 5

Breastfeeding and Gestational Diabetes

Renata Saucedo, Jorge Valencia, María Isabel Peña-Cano, Enrique Morales-Avila and Arturo Zárate

Abstract

Breastfeeding is recommended as the preferred method of feeding for infants for at least 1 year, because of its multiple immediate and long-term benefits for both the mother and child. Among women with a history of gestational diabetes mellitus (GDM), breastfeeding is associated with increased insulin sensitivity, improved insulin secretion, improved glucose tolerance, and a reduced incidence of type 2 diabetes mellitus (T2DM). Lactation has also been associated with postpartum weight loss, reduced long-term obesity risk, a lower prevalence of the metabolic syndrome, hypertension, and cardiovascular disease. The mechanisms underlying the benefits of breastfeeding for the mother are unclear. However, a role of adipose tissue-produced cytokines (adipokines) has been suggested. Lactation appears to mobilize adipose tissue accrued during pregnancy, and some changes in adipokine levels have been reported. Higher lactation intensity has been associated with lower plasma leptin, a peptide mainly associated with appetite regulation and insulin resistance.

Keywords: gestational diabetes, breastfeeding, leptin, insulin resistance, type 2 diabetes mellitus

1. Introduction

Breastmilk is the physiologic norm for infant nutrition, offering multiple health benefits and protection for babies and mothers [1–4]. WHO recommends that breastfeeding be initiated within 1 hour of birth, that it continue with no other foods or liquids for the first 6 months of life, and that it be continued with complementary feeding (breastfeeding with other age-appropriate foods) until at least 24 months of age. However, global breastfeeding rates remain far below international targets. In most high-income countries, the prevalence of breastfeeding at 12 months is lower than 20%, and it is highest in sub-Saharan Africa, south Asia, and parts of Latin America [5]. In Mexico, rates of breastfeeding are particularly low, 38.3% of Mexican women initiate breastfeeding soon after giving birth, only 14.4% of these women report exclusively breastfeeding at 6 months postpartum, 35.5% report any breastfeeding at 12 months postpartum, and 14.1% report any breastfeeding at 2 years postpartum. Importantly, breastfeeding rates vary by demographic area and are highest in rural over urban area [6].

Breastfeeding has protective effects on maternal health, including a reduced risk of breast cancer and ovarian cancer, obesity, hypertension, stroke, hyperlipidemia, metabolic syndrome, and type 2 diabetes mellitus (T2DM) [7–11].

One of the strongest risk factors for T2DM is a history of gestational diabetes mellitus (GDM). Among women with a history of GDM, the cumulative risk of developing T2DM at 10 years postpartum ranges from 20 to 50% [12]. Infant feeding method is a modifiable risk factor for the development of diabetes; breastfeeding confers short- and long-term benefits on metabolism reducing the risk of developing T2DM.

Despite the important benefits of breastfeeding, there is evidence to suggest that lower rates of breastfeeding occur in women with GDM and that the duration of breastfeeding is shorter compared with that of healthy mothers [13, 14]. The explanations to account for these rates are higher rates of cesarean sections and neonatal intensive care unit admissions, which include increased recovery time for the mother, prolonged separation of mother and baby, and decreased or delayed bonding [15]. Other factors influencing the lower rates of breastfeeding in GDM are insulin therapy during pregnancy and obesity; women with insulin-treated diabetes have less intention to breastfeed and women with high BMI may have different hormonal patterns, delaying onset of milk production [16, 17].

Insulin treatment is related to severity of GDM, and this marked gestational disturbance in insulin and glucose metabolism may interfere with the hormonal pathways for initiation of lactogenesis. Results from a study of gene expression profiles at different stages of lactation suggested that decreased insulin sensitivity may delay milk production as a result of protein tyrosine phosphatase, receptor type F overexpression in the mammary gland [18].

On the other hand, the GDM treatment with oral hypoglycemic agents has not been related to milk production by the mothers [16]. Glyburide and metformin are the two oral hypoglycemic agents most commonly used during pregnancy, and both are safe with breastfeeding [19].

2. Short-term benefits of breastfeeding

Lactation confers favorable metabolic changes, including lower fasting and postprandial blood glucose, as well as insulin, and triglycerides, and greater insulin sensitivity, and plasma HDL-C [20]. Glucose is diverted for milk production via noninsulin-mediated pathways of uptake by the mammary gland and, thus, lactating women exhibit lower blood glucose [21].

On the other hand, lactation promotes postpartum weight loss [22]; lactogenesis increases maternal total energy expenditure by 15–25% [23]. Prospective studies have reported more rapid weight loss within 6 months postpartum, and lower weight retention at 1 year postpartum [24].

Studies in women with recent GDM report more favorable glucose tolerance and lipid metabolism during 4 months postpartum for lactating compared with non-lactating women [25]. At 6–9 weeks postpartum, the SWIFT cohort in a racially and ethnically diverse group found a dose-response relationship between increasing intensity of lactation and decreasing fasting plasma glucose and both fasting and 2-h insulin, as well as improved insulin sensitivity [26].

In a retrospective cohort among Latinas with recent GDM, Kjos et al. reported 5 mg/dL lower fasting blood glucose for any intensity of lactation versus no lactation, and an improved glucose tolerance determined by the glucose area under the curve from the oral glucose tolerance test (OGTT) [27].

In a recent study of women with previous GDM diagnosed according to the new "International Association of Diabetes and Pregnancy Study Groups" (IADPSG) criteria, that included women with a milder metabolic impairment, breastfeeding for almost 3 months improved the metabolic outcomes, such as fasting and 2 h glycemia at OGTT, an index of insulin resistance (HOMA-IR) and triglycerides [28].

It has been demonstrated that the favorable effects of lactation on glucose metabolism persist after weaning. Chouinard-Castonguay et al., in a cross-sectional study, showed that lactation duration was an independent predictor of fasting insulin concentrations and insulin sensitivity indices up to a mean of 4 years after delivery [29].

3. Long-term benefits of breastfeeding

It has been suggested that a longer duration of breastfeeding is associated with a lower risk of T2DM. However, results in some studies have been inconsistent. Chouinard-Castonguay found that women who reported lactating for >10 months had impaired glucose tolerance less frequently compared with women who lactated for <10 months at 4 years postpartum [29].

In a longitudinal analysis, Buchanan found no difference in the prevalence of diabetes at 11–26 months postpartum [30]. Similarly, Kjos, in a retrospective study, reported that breastfeeding was not associated with the progression to T2DM within a follow-up of 7.5 years after delivery [27], and in a retrospective cohort study, the Nurses' Health Study, breastfeeding did not affect the risk of diabetes at 14 years [31].

However, of interest, one prospective study that assessed the development of T2DM in women with GDM for up to 20 years after delivery found that breastfeeding reduced the risk of diabetes by 46%; median time to postpartum diabetes was 12.3 years for women who breastfed versus 2.3 years for women who did not breastfeed, independently of maternal BMI and insulin use during pregnancy [32]. Moreover, women who breastfed for >3 months had lower risk of diabetes than women who breastfed for ≤3 months ($P = 0.029$).

Also, the positive metabolic impact of breastfeeding has been reported in women with mild forms of GDM. A recent study showed that women with glucose intolerance in early postpartum breastfed less often than women with a normal OGTT (69.5 vs. 84.2%, $p = 0.041$) [33].

The discrepancy among the different studies could be a result of the differences in the design of the study, the severity of GDM, diagnosis of T2DM, breastfeeding assessment, follow-up time postpartum sample size, lifestyle behaviors, ethnic characteristics, and, finally, the use of oral contraceptives. Birth control with progestin-only oral contraceptive pills has been associated with an increased risk of T2DM during the first 2 years of use. Kjos reported a threefold increase in the risk of T2DM at 7.5 years postpartum in breastfeeding women with recent GDM. By contrast, use of low dose progestin/estrogen combination oral contraceptive pills during breastfeeding does not increase the risk of T2DM [27].

4. Mechanisms in the protective effects of breastfeeding

The potential mechanisms involved in the protective effects of breastfeeding on glucose metabolism include breastfeeding-related hormones such as prolactin and estrogen [34]. Prolactin levels are elevated and estradiol is lower in breastfeeding women than in non-lactating women. In vitro experiments of rat pancreatic islets cultured with prolactin have shown enhanced stimulated insulin secretion through stimulation of b-cell proliferation by downregulating the expression of menin [35, 36]. Also, prolactin modulates the transcription factors STAT5 and PPARg, and the expression of lipoprotein lipase, which are co-expressed in breast, adipose tissue, and skeletal muscle [37].

On the other hand, it has been suggested that lactation improves insulin sensitivity by mobilizing lipids derived from liver and muscle for lactogenesis rather than by redirecting lipids into adipocytes [34].

Another mechanism is the influence of lactation on regional fat tissue metabolism; some studies have reported enhanced fat mass mobilization from the trunk and thighs for lactating women [38, 39]. In keeping with this, another study reported that lactation history is associated with a smaller visceral fat area in women who reported they lactated for at least 3 months [40].

There is also evidence that leptin, which is an adipokine positively associated with body adiposity and insulin resistance, is modified in breastfeeding women with previous GDM [41]. Leptin directly affects whole-body insulin sensitivity by regulating the efficiency of insulin-mediated glucose metabolism by skeletal muscle and by hepatic regulation of gluconeogenesis through its action on gene expression of phosphoenolpyruvate carboxykinase [42, 43]. Moreover, it exerts an acute inhibitory effect on insulin secretion, and upregulates inflammatory mediators like TNFα and interleukin-6, which contribute to excessive insulin resistance both at the level of the whole body and in specific organs, including in the liver, muscle, and brain [44].

Leptin is predominantly produced by adipocytes, but is also produced by non-adipose tissues such as stomach, intestine, ovaries, and in particular, the placenta [45]. Maternal leptin levels increase two- to threefold in pregnancy, with a peak occurring around 28 weeks of gestation and decreasing to pre-pregnancy concentrations after delivery [46]. It has been suggested that the rise in maternal leptin concentration during pregnancy may result from an upregulation of adipocyte leptin synthesis in the presence of increasing insulin resistance and hyperinsulinemia in the second half of pregnancy [47]. However, there is strong evidence that the placenta, rather than maternal adipose tissue, contributes to the increase of maternal leptin concentrations during pregnancy [48]. Leptin induces human chorionic gonadotropin production, regulates placental growth, angiogenesis, trophoblast invasion, and nutrient transfer [49]. Leptin enhances the mobilization of maternal fat stores to increase availability and to support transplacental transfer of lipid substrates [50]. Moreover, leptin upregulates placental System A amino acid transport, to increase fetal nutrient availability [51]. Leptin serves as a mitogen for a growing number of cell types, including endothelial cells, hemopoietic cells, lung epithelial cells, and pancreatic b-cells in vitro [52]. Leptin could therefore be stimulating growth of tissues in the developing fetus.

Leptin contributes to the pathophysiologic relationship between GDM and subsequent T2DM. In our previous study, we found that women with previous GDM persisted with insulin resistance in the postpartum period, in association with higher leptin levels compared with the control group [53]. It is possible that postpartum insulin resistance may be contributing to these elevated levels. A positive association between leptinemia and insulinemia has been reported in numerous studies of obese and non-obese humans [54, 55]. Experimentally, increased insulin levels may stimulate leptin production in adipocytes, and vice versa, an increase in leptin levels may lead to insulin resistance and alter b-cell secretory capacity [56, 57]. Interestingly, we recently reported that breastfeeding was associated with better metabolic profile in the early postpartum period in women with previous

GDM, showing that women with longer duration of lactation had greater weight loss at postpartum and lower leptin levels compared with women who lactated for a short period. This difference remained statistically significant after adjustment for weight [58]. Similarly, a previous study with a large cohort of women with recent GDM that utilized a quantitative measure of lactation intensity found that mean leptin concentrations were inversely associated with lactation intensity (lower by 15–21%) independent of maternal pre-pregnancy obesity, race, weight loss, sociodemographics, and postpartum insulin resistance [41]. It has been suggested that during lactation, prolactin suppresses leptin secretion [59].

On the other hand, leptin is a long-term regulator of appetite that serves as an anorexigenic signal when adipose stores are high [60]. It has been detected in breast milk at concentrations of 0.35–4.6 μg/L [61], and the concentration of leptin in breast milk is correlated to indices of maternal adiposity, including body mass index ($r = 0.65$, $P < 0.02$), and fat mass ($r = 0.65$, $P < 0.02$) [62]. This evidence provides an attractive explanation for the ability of breast milk to regulate infant body weight. Bouret has recently suggested that the presence of appetite hormones may permanently affect the appetite-regulating system of the infant by affecting the development of the hypothalamus. These differences in appetite hormone exposure may create permanent changes in the way the brain reacts to appetite hormones and satiety cues [63].

Another adipokine related to abnormal glucose metabolism during pregnancy is adiponectin. It has been suggested that low levels of adiponectin may induce severe insulin resistance prior to the onset of GDM [64]. Gunderson evaluated the relationship between lactation intensity and plasma adiponectin among postpartum women with previous GDM and found that higher lactation intensity was associated with 6% lower adiponectin. This inverse association remained after adjustment for insulin resistance [41]. This observation is consistent with the action of prolactin in suppressing the production and secretion of adiponectin from human adipocytes [13].

5. Implications of breastfeeding in the offspring of the GDM mother

Infants of mothers with GDM are at increased risk of prematurity, macrosomia, hypoglycemia, respiratory distress, hypocalcemia, polycythemia, and hyperbilirubinemia. Breastfeeding has many established benefits for child health; it prevents child morbidity due to diarrhea, respiratory infections, and otitis media [5]. In particular, in the offspring of the GDM mother, lactation has been associated with lower episodes of hypoglycemia [65].

On the other hand, exposure to maternal gestational diabetes has been shown to increase the risk of obesity, childhood-onset type 2 diabetes in offspring, as well as the risk of adult-onset type 2 diabetes and gestational diabetes in those offspring [66]. Breastfeeding confers protection against these medical complications; exclusive breastfeeding decreases the risk of the development of childhood-onset type 2 diabetes and obesity [67].

Benefits of breastfeeding on children's health are likely due to the unique composition of breast milk. Human milk is a source of immunoglobulins, hormones and growth factors including leptin, adiponectin, ghrelin, peptide YY, glucagon-like peptide-1, resistin, and obestatin, which are involved in food intake regulation and energy balance, and may have a role in the regulation of growth and development in the neonatal period and infancy, as well as long-term effects on metabolic programming [68].

6. Suggestions for mothers with GDM regarding breastfeeding

Women whose pregnancy is affected by GDM should be educated early as to the benefits of breastfeeding their offspring. An increase in breastfeeding duration among women with GDM has been demonstrated with prenatal education. Breastfeeding support in the hospital immediately after delivery and during the postpartum period as well as community support that encourages breastfeeding are also essential. Electronic alerts via text message or email, automated letters, and nurse phone contact may increase uptake. This targeted breastfeeding support for women with GDM is feasible and efficacious, and could be integrated into GDM management [69].

Likewise, insulin treatment during pregnancy should be considered a targeting indicator for providing extra skilled breastfeeding support to GDM women who decide to breastfeed [16].

7. Conclusions

Breastfeeding is recommended and encouraged for mothers, as it has multiple benefits for both women and children. Mothers who breastfeed have been shown to have reduced risk of developing subsequent breast cancer and ovarian cancer, obesity, hypertension, stroke, hyperlipidemia, metabolic syndrome, and T2DM. In women with GDM, several studies suggest that breastfeeding is associated with reduced risk of T2DM. Despite this important benefit, there is evidence to suggest that lower rates of breastfeeding occur in women with GDM. Evidence has shown that healthcare provider support of breastfeeding along with patient education has a significant impact on breastfeeding rates. The medical and behavioral communities should be better able to design, implement, and administer public health programs that may promote healthy lifestyle behaviors including breastfeeding among GDM women, and mitigating T2DM risk.

Acknowledgements

RS holds a fellowship from the National System of Investigators. We thank the Hospital of Gynecology and Obstetrics, Medical Center La Raza, Instituto Mexicano del Seguro Social, for providing patient care services.

This work was supported by scientific grants from IMSS.

Conflict of interest

The authors declare that there is no conflict of interests regarding the publication of this chapter.

Thanks

This chapter is dedicated to the memory of Dr. Arturo Zárate (1936–2018), pioneer in the field of Gynecological Endocrinology in Mexico.

Author details

Renata Saucedo[1]*, Jorge Valencia[1], María Isabel Peña-Cano[2], Enrique Morales-Avila[2] and Arturo Zárate[1]

1 Endocrine Research Unit, National Medical Center, Instituto Mexicano del Seguro Social, Mexico City, Mexico

2 Faculty of Chemistry, Universidad Autonoma del Estado de Mexico, State of Mexico, Mexico

*Address all correspondence to: sgrenata@yahoo.com

References

[1] Bartick MC, Stuebe AM, Schwarz EB, Luongo C, Reinhold AG, Foster EM. Cost analysis of maternal disease associated with suboptimal breastfeeding. Obstetrics and Gynecology. 2013;**122**:111-119. DOI: 10.1097/AOG.0b013e318297a047

[2] Gunderson EP, Lewis CE, Wei GS, Whitmer RA, Quesenberry CP, Sidney S. Lactation and changes in maternal metabolic risk factors. Obstetrics and Gynecology. 2007;**109**:729-738

[3] Hanson LA. Human milk and host defence: Immediate and long-term effects. Acta Paediatrica Supplement. 1999;**88**:42-46

[4] Plagemann A, Harder T. Breastfeeding and the risk of obesity and related metabolic diseases in the child. Metabolic Syndrome and Related Disorders. 2005;**3**:222-232. DOI: 10.1089/met.2005.3.222

[5] Victora CG, Bahl R, Barros AJ, França GV, Horton S, Krasevec J, et al. Breastfeeding in the 21st century: Epidemiology, mechanisms, and lifelong effect. Lancet. 2016;**387**: 475-490. DOI: 10.1016/S0140-6736(15) 01024-7

[6] Gutiérrez JP, Rivera-Domarco J, Shamah-Levy T, Villalpando-Hernández S, Franco A, Cuevas-Nasu L, et al. Encuesta Nacional de Salud y Nutrición 2012. Resultados Nacionales. Cuernavaca, México: Instituto Nacional de Salud Pública (MX); 2012

[7] Bernier MO, Plu-Bureau G, Bossard N, Ayzac L, Thalabard JC. Breastfeeding and risk of breast cancer: A metaanalysis of published studies. Human Reproduction Update. 2000;**6**:374-386

[8] Danforth KN, Tworoger SS, Hecht JL, Rosner BA, Colditz GA, Hankinson SE. Breastfeeding and risk of ovarian cancer in two prospective cohorts. Cancer Causes & Control. 2007;**18**: 517-523

[9] Stuebe AM, Schwarz EB, Grewen K, Rich-Edwards JW, Michels KB, Foster EM, et al. Duration of lactation and incidence of maternal hypertension: A longitudinal cohort study. American Journal of Epidemiology. 2011;**174**: 1147-1158. DOI: 10.1093/aje/kwr227

[10] Schwarz EB, Ray RM, Stuebe AM, Allison MA, Ness RB, Freiberg MS, et al. Duration of lactation and risk factors for maternal cardiovascular disease. Obstetrics and Gynecology. 2009;**113**: 974-982. DOI: 10.1097/01. AOG.0000346884.67796.ca

[11] Jacobson LT, Hade EM, Collins TC, Margolis KL, Waring ME, Van Horn LV, et al. Breastfeeding history and risk of stroke among parous postmenopausal women in the Women's Health Initiative. Journal of the American Heart Association. 2018;**7**:e008739. DOI: 10.1161/JAHA.118.008739

[12] Bellamy L, Casas JP, Hingorani AD, Williams D. Type 2 diabetes mellitus after gestational diabetes: A systematic review and meta-analysis. Lancet. 2009; **373**:1773-1779. DOI: 10.1016/ S0140-6736(09)60731-5

[13] Asai-Sato M, Okamoto M, Endo M, Yoshida H, Murase M, Ikeda M, et al. Hypoadiponectinemia in lean lactating women: Prolactin inhibits adiponectin secretion from human adipocytes. Endocrine Journal. 2006;**53**:555-562

[14] Hummel S, Hummel M, Knopff A, Bonifacio E, Ziegler AG. Breastfeeding in women with gestational diabetes. Deutsche Medizinische Wochenschrift. 2008;**133**:180-184. DOI: 10.1055/s-2008-1017493

[15] Soltani H, Arden M. Factors associated with breastfeeding up to 6 months postpartum in mothers with diabetes. Journal of Obstetric, Gynecologic, and Neonatal Nursing. 2009;**38**:586-594

[16] Matias SL, Dewey KG, Quesenberry CP Jr, Gunderson EP. Maternal prepregnancy obesity and insulin treatment during pregnancy are independently associated with delayed lactogenesis in women with recent gestational diabetes mellitus. The American Journal of Clinical Nutrition. 2014;**99**:115-121. DOI: 10.3945/ajcn.113.073049

[17] Finkelstein SA, Keely E, Feig DS, Tu X, Yasseen AS III, Walker M. Breastfeeding in women with diabetes: Lower rates despite greater rewards. A population-based study. Diabetic Medicine. 2013;**30**:1094-1101

[18] Lemay DG, Ballard OA, Hughes MA, Morrow AL, Horseman ND, Nommsen-Rivers LA. RNA sequencing of the human milk fat layer transcriptome reveals distinct gene expression profiles at three stages of lactation. PLoS One. 2013;**8**:e67531. DOI: 10.1371/journal.pone.0067531

[19] Refuerzo JS. Oral hypoglycemic agents in pregnancy. Obstetrics and Gynecology Clinics of North America. 2011;**38**:227-234. DOI: 10.1016/j.ogc.2011.02.013

[20] Stuebe A. Associations among lactation, maternal carbohydrate metabolism, and cardiovascular health. Clinical Obstetrics and Gynecology. 2015;**58**:827-839. DOI: 10.1097/GRF.0000000000000155

[21] Bell AW, Bauman DE. Adaptations of glucose metabolism during pregnancy and lactation. Journal of Mammary Gland Biology and Neoplasia. 1997;**2**:265-278

[22] Baker JL, Gamborg M, Heitmann BL, Lissner L, Sørensen TI, Rasmussen KM. Breastfeeding reduces postpartum weight retention. The American Journal of Clinical Nutrition. 2008;**88**:1543-1551. DOI: 10.3945/ajcn.2008.26379

[23] Butte NF, Hopkinson JM, Mehta N, Moon JK, Smith EO. Adjustments in energy expenditure and substrate utilization during late pregnancy and lactation. The American Journal of Clinical Nutrition. 1999;**69**:299-307

[24] Janney CA, Zhang D, Sowers M. Lactation and weight retention. The American Journal of Clinical Nutrition. 1997;**66**:1116-1124

[25] Gunderson EP. Impact of breastfeeding on maternal metabolism: Implications for women with gestational diabetes. Current Diabetes Reports. 2014;**14**:460. DOI: 10.1007/s11892-013-0460-2

[26] Gunderson EP, Hedderson MM, Chiang V, Crites Y, Walton D, Azevedo RA, et al. Lactation intensity and postpartum maternal glucose tolerance and insulin resistance in women with recent GDM: The SWIFT cohort. Diabetes Care. 2012;**35**:50-56. DOI: 10.2337/dc11-1409

[27] Kjos SL, Peters RK, Xiang A, Thomas D, Schaefer U, Buchanan TA. Contraception and the risk of type 2 diabetes mellitus in Latina women with prior gestational diabetes mellitus. Journal of the American Medical Association. 1998;**280**:533-538

[28] Corrado F, Giunta L, Granese R, Corrado S, Micali M, Santamaria A, et al. Metabolic effects of breastfeeding in women with previous gestational diabetes diagnosed according to the IADPSG criteria. The Journal of Maternal-Fetal & Neonatal Medicine. 2017;**19**:1-4. DOI: 10.1080/14767058.2017.1377175

[29] Chouinard-Castonguay S, Weisnagel SJ, Tchernof A, Robitaille J. Relationship between lactation duration and insulin and glucose response among women with prior gestational diabetes. European Journal of Endocrinology. 2013;**168**:515-523. DOI: 10.1530/EJE-12-0939

[30] Buchanan TA, Xiang AH, Kjos SL, Trigo E, Lee WP, Peters RK. Antepartum predictors of the development of type 2 diabetes in Latino women 11-26 months after pregnancies complicated by gestational diabetes. Diabetes. 1999;**48**:2430-2436

[31] Stuebe AM, Rich-Edwards JW, Willett WC, Manson JE, Michels KB. Duration of lactation and incidence of type 2 diabetes. Journal of the American Medical Association. 2005;**294**: 2601-2610

[32] Ziegler AG, Wallner M, Kaiser I, Rossbauer M, Harsunen MH, Lachmann L, et al. Long-term protective effect of lactation on the development of type 2 diabetes in women with recent gestational diabetes mellitus. Diabetes. 2012;**61**:3167-3171. DOI: 10.2337/db12-0393

[33] Benhalima K, Jegers K, Devlieger R, Verhaeghe J, Mathieu C. Glucose intolerance after a recent history of gestational diabetes based on the 2013 WHO criteria. PLoS One. 2016;**11**: e0157272. DOI: 10.1371/journal.pone.0157272

[34] Much D, Beyerlein A, Roßbauer M, Hummel S, Ziegler AG. Beneficial effects of breastfeeding in women with gestational diabetes mellitus. Molecular Metabolism. 2014;**3**:284-292. DOI: 10.1016/j.molmet.2014.01.002

[35] Crepaldi SC, Carneiro EM, Boschero AC. Long-term effect of prolactin treatment on glucose-induced insulin secretion in cultured neonatal rat islets. Hormone and Metabolic Research. 1997; **29**:220-224

[36] Karnik SK, Chen H, McLean GW, Heit JJ, Gu X, Zhang AY, et al. Menin controls growth of pancreatic beta-cells in pregnant mice and promotes gestational diabetes mellitus. Science. 2007;**318**:806-809

[37] Ramos-Román MA. Prolactin and lactation as modifiers of diabetes risk in gestational diabetes. Hormone and Metabolic Research. 2011;**43**:593-600. DOI: 10.1055/s-0031-1284353

[38] Sohlström A, Forsum E. Changes in adipose tissue volume and distribution during reproduction in Swedish women as assessed by magnetic resonance imaging. The American Journal of Clinical Nutrition. 1995;**61**:287-295

[39] Forsum E, Sadurskis A, Wager J. Estimation of body fat in healthy Swedish women during pregnancy and lactation. The American Journal of Clinical Nutrition. 1989;**50**:465-473

[40] McClure CK, Catov J, Ness R, Schwarz EB. Maternal visceral adiposity by consistency of lactation. Maternal and Child Health Journal. 2012;**16**: 316-321. DOI: 10.1007/s10995-011-0758-0

[41] Gunderson EP, Kim C, Quesenberry CP Jr, Marcovina S, Walton D, Azevedo RA, et al. Lactation intensity and fasting plasma lipids, lipoproteins, non-esterified free fatty acids, leptin and adiponectin in postpartum women with recent gestational diabetes mellitus: The SWIFT cohort. Metabolism. 2014;**63**: 941-950. DOI: 10.1016/j.metabol.2014.04.006

[42] Saucedo R, Valencia J, Gutierrez C, Zárate A. The role of leptin in gestational diabetes mellitus. In: Gilles E, Mickaël D, editors. Leptin: Production, Regulation and Functions.

New York: Nova Science Publishers, Inc; 2017. pp. 131-150

[43] Rossetti L, Massillon D, Barzilai N, Vuguin P, Chen W, Hawkins M. Short term effects of leptin on hepatic gluconeogenesis and in vivo insulin action. The Journal of Biological Chemistry. 1997;**272**:27758-27763

[44] Ouchi N, Parker JL, Lugus JJ, Walsh K. Adipokines in inflammation and metabolic disease. Nature Reviews Immunology. 2011;**11**:85-97

[45] Ashworth CJ, Hoggard N, Thomas L, Mercer JG, Wallace JM, Lea RG. Placental leptin. Reviews of Reproduction. 2000;**5**:18-24

[46] Schubring C, Englaroe P, Sieblerb T, Blumd WF, Demirakcad T, Kratzschc J, et al. Longitudinal analysis of maternal serum leptin levels during pregnancy, at birth and up to six weeks after birth: Relation to body mass index, skinfolds, sex steroids and umbilical cord blood leptin levels. Hormone Research. 1998; **50**:276-283

[47] Laivuori H, Kaaja R, Koistinen H, Karonen SL, Andersson S, Koivisto V, et al. Leptin during and after preeclamptic or normal pregnancy: Its relation to serum insulin and insulin sensitivity. Metabolism. 2000;**49**: 259-263

[48] Masuzaki H, Ogawa Y, Sagawa N, Hosoda K, Matsumoto T, Mise H, et al. Nonadipose tissue production of leptin: Leptin as a novel placenta-derived hormone in humans. Nature Medicine. 1997;**3**:1029-1033

[49] Sagawa N, Yura S, Itoh H, Kakui K, Takemura M, Nuamah MA, et al. Possible role of placental leptin in pregnancy: A review. Endocrine. 2002;**19**:65-71

[50] Sattar N, Greer IA, Pirwani I, Gibson J, Wallace AM. Leptin levels in pregnancy: Marker for fat accumulation and mobilization? Acta Obstetricia et Gynecologica Scandinavica. 1998;**77**: 278-283

[51] Jansson N, Greenwood SL, Johansson BR, Powell TL, Jansson T. Leptin stimulates the activity of the system A amino acid transporter in human placental villous fragments. The Journal of Clinical Endocrinology and Metabolism. 2003;**88**:1205-1211

[52] Christou H, Serdy S, Mantzoros CS. Leptin in relation to growth and developmental processes in the fetus. Seminars in Reproductive Medicine. 2002;**20**:23-130

[53] Saucedo R, Zarate A, Basurto L, Hernandez M, Puello E, Galvan R, et al. Relationship between circulating adipokines and insulin resistance during pregnancy and pospartum in women with gestational diabetes. Archives of Medical Research. 2011;**42**:318-323

[54] Saad MF, Khan A, Sharma A. Physiological insulinemia acutely modulates plasma leptin. Diabetes. 1998;**47**:544-549

[55] Utriainen T, Malmstroem R, Maekimattila S. Supraphysiological hyperinsulinemia increases plasma leptin concentrations after 4 h in normal subjects. Diabetes. 1996;**45**: 1364-1366

[56] Zeigerer A, Rodeheffer MS, McGraw TE. Insulin regulates leptin secretion from 3T3eL1 adipocytes by a PI 3 kinase independent mechanism. Experimental Cell Research. 2008;**314**: 2249-2256

[57] Kieffer TJ, Habener JF. The adipoinsular axis: Effects of leptin on pancreatic beta-cells. American Journal of Physiology: Endocrinology and Metabolism. 2000;**278**:E1-E14

[58] Saucedo R, Basurto L, Galván R, Sánchez J, Puello E, Zárate A. Duration of lactation is associated with lower leptin levels in patients with gestational diabetes mellitus. Salud(i)Ciencia. 2014; **20**:581-585

[59] Feuermann Y, Mabjeesh SJ, Niv-Spector L, Levin D, Shamay A. Prolactin affects leptin action in the bovine mammary gland via the mammary fat pad. The Journal of Endocrinology. 2006;**191**:407-413

[60] Halaas JL, Gajiwala KS, Maffei M, Cohen SL, Chait BT, Rabinowitz D, et al. Weight-reducing effects of the plasma protein encoded by the obese gene. Science. 1995;**269**:543-546

[61] Casabiell X, Piñeiro V, Tomé MA, Peinó R, Diéguez C, Casanueva FF. Presence of leptin in colostrum and/or breast milk from lactating mothers: A potential role in the regulation of neonatal food intake. The Journal of Clinical Endocrinology and Metabolism. 1997;**82**:4270-4273

[62] Schueler J, Alexander B, Hart AM, Austin K, Larson-Meyer DE. Presence and dynamics of leptin, GLP-1, and PYY in human breast milk at early postpartum. Obesity. 2013;**21**:1451-1458. DOI: 10.1002/oby.20345

[63] Bouret SG. Early life origins of obesity: Role of hypothalamic programming. Journal of Pediatric Gastroenterology and Nutrition. 2009; **48**(Supp. 1):S31-S38. DOI: 10.1097/MPG.0b013e3181977375

[64] Retnakaran R, Hanley AJ, Raif N, Connelly PW, Sermer M, Zinman B. Reduced adiponectin concentration in women with gestational diabetes: A potential factor in progression to type 2 diabetes. Diabetes Care. 2004;**27**: 799-800

[65] Cordero L, Treuer SH, Landon MB, Gabbe SG. Management of infants of diabetic mothers. Archives of Pediatrics & Adolescent Medicine. 1998;**152**: 249-254

[66] Dabelea D. The predisposition to obesity and diabetes in offspring of diabetic mothers. Diabetes Care. 2007; **30**(Supp. 2):S169-S174. DOI: 10.2337/dc07-s211

[67] Halipchuk J, Temple B, Dart A, Martin D, Sellers EAC. Prenatal, obstetric and perinatal factors associated with the development of childhood-onset type 2 diabetes. Canadian Journal of Diabetes. 2018;**42**:71-77. DOI: 10.1016/j.jcjd.2017.04.003

[68] Savino F, Benetti S, Liguori SA, Sorrenti M, Cordero Di Montezemolo L. Advances on human milk hormones and protection against obesity. Cellular and Molecular Biology. 2013;**59**:89-98

[69] Stuebe AM, Bonuck K, Adatorwovor R, Schwartz TA, Berry DC. A cluster randomized trial of tailored breastfeeding support for women with gestational diabetes. Breastfeeding Medicine. 2016;**11**: 504-513

Section 3

Current Concepts

Chapter 6

Screening for Gestational Diabetes Mellitus: The Potential of MicroRNAs

Carmen Pheiffer, Stephanie Dias, Paul Rheeder and Sumaiya Adam

Abstract

Gestational diabetes mellitus (GDM) is associated with short- and long-term complications in both mothers and their offspring. Screening and early diagnosis of GDM is advocated as a strategy to prevent adverse pregnancy outcomes. However, there is currently no test that is amenable to routine screening, particularly in low-and middle-income countries. MicroRNAs (miRNAs) are small non-coding RNA molecules that regulate gene expression post-transcriptionally. In recent years, miRNAs have been the focus of increasing research due to their important role in regulating biological pathways and their aberrant expression during disease. The discovery of circulating miRNAs in maternal blood, and their altered expression during pregnancy-associated complications have increased interest into their potential as diagnostic biomarkers for GDM. In this review, we summarise studies that have investigated miRNAs in maternal blood thus providing an update of the current status of miRNAs as biomarkers for GDM. We also discuss the challenges of miRNA profiling, and highlight perspectives and recommendations for research.

Keywords: gestational diabetes mellitus, biomarkers, epigenetics, microRNAs, pregnancy

1. Introduction

Gestational diabetes mellitus (GDM) is defined as glucose intolerance that is first diagnosed during pregnancy with glucose homeostasis usually restored shortly after birth. The rate of GDM has constantly increased over the last 20 years [1], and in 2017 the International Diabetes Federation estimated that about 14% of women with live births had GDM [2]. Without appropriate glucose management, GDM is associated with short- and long-term complications in both mothers and their offspring [3–6]. Treatment of GDM is effective in preventing these adverse outcomes [7–11], thus, universal screening and early detection of GDM is widely advocated as a strategy to promote timely treatment and improve pregnancy outcomes [3]. The oral glucose tolerance test (OGTT) conducted between the 24th and 28th week of pregnancy, is currently the gold standard for GDM diagnosis [12]. However, the test is time-consuming, expensive and unfeasible in most countries. The identification of simple and cost-effective biomarkers that do not require fasting and multiple blood draws would be more acceptable to pregnant women, and thereby facilitate screening for GDM. MicroRNAs (miRNAs) are small noncoding RNA molecules that regulate various metabolic pathways. They are implicated in the pathophysiology of various diseases and have attracted considerable interest as biomarkers of metabolic disease. Recently, several studies have explored their potential as biomarkers of GDM. The purpose of this review is to provide an update of the status of miRNAs as biomarkers for GDM. All studies that have profiled miRNAs in maternal blood during GDM to date are summarised. We also discuss the challenges of miRNA research, and highlight perspectives and recommendations for future research.

2. Overview of gestational diabetes

Hyperglycaemia during pregnancy creates an adverse intrauterine environment that predisposes both mother and offspring to perinatal complications and future metabolic disease [3–6]. Maternal perinatal complications include caesarean section, preeclampsia and birth injuries. Women with pregnancies complicated by GDM also have an increased risk of developing disease in later life. In 2009, Bellamy et al. conducted a comprehensive review of the literature and found that women who have had GDM are at least seven-fold more likely to develop Type 2 diabetes (T2D) compared to women with normoglycaemic pregnancies [4]. Other studies showed that GDM is associated with the development of metabolic disease [13], cardiovascular disease [14] and breast cancer [15].

Foetal and neonatal complications associated with GDM include macrosomia, congenital malformations, perinatal death, hypertrophic cardiomyopathy, intrauterine growth restriction, preterm birth, respiratory distress syndrome, hypoglycaemia, hypocalcaemia, polycythaemia and hyperbilirubinemia [5]. In recent years, increasing evidence support the critical role of the intrauterine environment in programming the foetus and influencing long-term offspring health [16]. In the 1980s, David Barker and his colleagues proposed *Barker's hypothesis* or *the developmental origins of adult disease*, which suggests that metabolic diseases have their origins in early development [17]. Subsequently, several other studies have reported that diabetes during pregnancy is associated with the development of obesity and diabetes in children [5].

The prevalence of GDM is rapidly increasing, spurred by the global obesity pandemic. Pregnant women who are overweight, obese or severely obese have a 2.14-, 3.56- and 8.56-fold risk of developing GDM compared to normal weight women [18]. The short- and long-term consequences of GDM are likely to have a major negative impact, particularly on low- and middle-income countries that already have limited financial and human resources, and are least able to respond to the challenge. Screening and treatment of GDM leads to improved pregnancy outcomes [7–11], thus universal screening for GDM is widely advocated as a strategy to prevent pregnancy complications. However, the OGTT, which is considered the gold standard for GDM diagnosis is not amenable to routine screening [3]. Currently, traditional risk-factor screening based on obesity, age older than ≥35 years, non-white ethnicity, and having a family history of diabetes [3] is mostly employed. Unfortunately, these risk factors have poor predictive value [19, 20]. A number of other laboratory tests such as glycated haemoglobin (HbA1c), insulin, adiponectin, glycosylated fibronectin and C-reactive protein have been explored, however, they too have several challenges and are not yet clinically applicable [3].

3. Characteristics of ideal biomarkers

Biomarkers are defined as "cellular, biochemical or molecular alterations that are measurable in biological media such as human tissues, cells or fluids" [21].

Screening, diagnostic and prognostic biomarkers offer several advantages and thus efforts to identify biomarkers of disease have intensified. They are clinically useful and can be used to detect or monitor disease progression, thus facilitating earlier diagnosis and disease management. Furthermore, biomarkers are able to monitor pharmacological responses and predict clinical outcome. As recently reviewed by Etheridge et al. [22], characteristics of the ideal biomarker include sensitivity, specificity, cost-effectiveness, reproducibility, robustness, accessibility, stability and ability to differentiate between pathologies. Recent advancements in molecular biology have led to the development of molecular biomarkers that are sensitive and specific, and are easily measured in biological fluids such as whole blood, plasma and serum [22].

4. MicroRNAs

MiRNAs are epigenetic mechanisms that reflect gene-environment interactions and are increasingly being implicated in the pathophysiology of metabolic diseases [23]. Since their discovery in *Caenorhabditis elegans* in 1993 [24], miRNAs have emerged as one of the most powerful epigenetic mechanisms regulating diverse biological processes including development, proliferation, differentiation and apoptosis [25]. They are short, single-stranded, highly conserved, non-coding RNA molecules of approximately 22 nucleotides in length that regulate gene expression through post-transcriptional mechanisms. MiRNAs bind to the 3′ untranslated region (UTR) of messenger RNA (mRNA) inducing degradation or translational repression of the mRNA transcript [26]. Using an elegant set of experiments, Guo et al. showed that destabilisation of target mRNAs rather than translational repression is the main mechanism whereby miRNAs reduce protein expression [26]. A single miRNA is able to regulate up to 200 target genes, implying that about 30% of the genome is regulated by miRNAs [27, 28] and confirming the important role of miRNAs as mediators of biological function. More than 2000 miRNAs are present in the human genome, and function in various biological processes [27–29].

Mature miRNAs are produced through a stepwise process. Briefly, primary miRNA transcripts (pri-miRNAs) are transcribed in the nucleus by RNA polymerase II (and possibly by RNA polymerase III), which are then cleaved by Drosha RNase III endonuclease to produce stem-loop precursor miRNAs (pre-miRNAs) that are approximately 70 nucleotides long. Ran-GTP and the export receptor, Exportin-5 transports pre-miRNAs to the cytoplasm, where Dicer, also a RNase III endonuclease, cleaves them to produce mature miRNAs. Mature miRNAs complex with the RNA-induced silencing complex (RISC) and bind to the 3' UTR of mRNA to induce predominantly mRNA degradation [25, 26].

MiRNAs regulate a wide range of biological processes including cell proliferation and differentiation, apoptosis and metabolism, thus it is not surprising that altered miRNA expression have been shown to associated with various conditions including cancer, obesity, T2D and cardiovascular disease [30]. MiRNAs play a critical role in the pathophysiology of metabolic disease, and their aberrant expression is observed in tissues associated with disease. For example, various *in vitro*, *in vivo* animal models and studies in diabetic patients have demonstrated the altered expression of miRNAs that regulate insulin secretion, adipocyte differentiation, lipid metabolism, inflammation and glucose homeostasis in dysfunctional pancreatic beta cells and insulin-resistant target tissues, such as adipose, liver and muscle during T2D [23]. Increasingly evidence show that correcting aberrant miRNA expression can prevent or treat T2D, making them attractive therapeutic targets [31].

The identification of circulating miRNAs in biological fluids such as whole blood, serum, plasma and urine has sparked research efforts to investigate their feasibility as diagnostic or prognostic biomarkers of disease [32–34]. Circulating miRNAs are speculated to reflect tissue expression, to play a central role in cell-to-cell communication and to be associated with disease progression [33–35]. Other attributes that make miRNAs attractive biomarkers is their stability and robust expression [22], even in degraded RNA samples [36]. Technological advances and the development of various platforms for miRNA profiling have bolstered the popularity of miRNAs [37], and have enabled relative easy and cost-effective methods of quantification using sensitive techniques such as quantitative real time PCR (qRT-PCR) [22, 32, 38]. Circulating miRNAs are thought to be released from cells as exosomes, microvesicles, apoptotic bodies, or are non-vesicle bound and encapsulated in protein or lipid complexes [32]. A number of studies [39–41], have demonstrated that circulating miRNAs are associated with glucose homeostasis and are dysregulated during T2D progression. Recently, we showed that the expression of miR-27b is increased in peripheral blood cells and serum of South African women with impaired glucose tolerance compared to normoglycaemia [42] and identified novel miRNAs associated with dysglycaemia in these women [43]. Putative gene targets of these novel miRNAs were enriched in biological processes involved in key aspects of glucose regulation, and receiver operating characteristic (ROC) curve analysis demonstrated that the diagnostic utility of these miRNAs were similar to fasting insulin [43]. Intriguingly, Parrizas et al. showed that an exercise intervention was able to reverse the aberrant expression of miR-192 and miR-193b induced by impaired glucose tolerance [44], while Luo et al. [45] showed that platelet-derived miR-126 was altered during T2D progression, and that glucose lowering treatment was able to normalise its expression. These studies provide support for the use of miRNAs as diagnostic and prognostic biomarkers to monitor treatment response.

5. MicroRNAs, pregnancy and gestational diabetes

MiRNAs play an important role as metabolic and developmental regulators during pregnancy. They respond to changing physiological conditions during pregnancy, while their dysregulation contributes to pregnancy-related disorders [46]. Thus far over 600 placental miRNAs have been identified [47]. Altered placental miRNA expression has been demonstrated in several pregnancy related disorders. In 2007, Pineles et al. were the first to demonstrate altered miRNA expression during preeclampsia. They reported that the expression of two miRNAs, miR-210 and miR-182, were increased during preeclampsia [48]. In 2009, using microarrays, Hu et al. and Zhu et al. identified seven and 34 miRNAs, respectively, that are dysregulated in preeclamptic compared to normal pregnancies [49, 50]. Subsequently, other studies have reported differential miRNA expression during preeclampsia and importantly provide experimental evidence to support the involvement of these miRNAs in disease pathophysiology [51, 52]. Altered miRNA expression has also been observed in other pregnancy complications such as macrosomia [53], preterm delivery and small for gestational age [54].

Placental-derived miRNAs in maternal blood have potential as biomarkers for pregnancy monitoring [54, 55]. It is suggested that miRNAs from placental tissue are exported into the maternal circulation via exosomes, and that these miRNAs reflect the physiological status of pregnancy and may thus have diagnostic potential [56]. Many of studies have reported that maternal circulating miRNAs are associated with placental weight [57], placental dysfunction [58, 59] and pregnancy complications [54, 60–63]. MiR-517c was increased in pregnancies complicated with placental abruption [59], miR-515, miR-516a, miR-516b, miR-518b, miR-519d, miR-520a, miR-520h, miR-525, miR-526b and miR-1323 were increased during preeclampsia [63], miR-516, miR-517, miR-520a, miR-525 and miR-526a were upregulated during preeclampsia, gestational hypertension and foetal growth restriction [60], miR-517a was increased and miR-518b was decreased during placenta previa [58], and miR-346 and miR-582 were increased during preeclampsia, preterm delivery and small for gestational age patients compared to normal controls [54]. Importantly, Hromadnikova et al. showed that upregulation of plasma miR-517, miR-518b and miR-520h during the first trimester was associated with the development of preeclampsia, and provided evidence to suggest that miR-517 could predict preeclampsia [61]. Furthermore, a number of studies have reported that circulating miRNAs are associated with macrosomia [62, 64, 65]. Jiang and colleagues demonstrated that maternal expression of miR-21, and to a lesser extent miR-20a in serum samples from pregnant women in the third trimester was associated with macrosomia [62], Hu et al. reported that macrosomia was associated with decreased serum expression of miR-376a [64], while Ge et al. reported that the expression of miR-18a, miR-141, miR-143, miR-200c and miR-221 were decreased, and miR-16, miR-30a and miR-523 were increased in the plasma of pregnant women with foetal macrosomia compared to normal controls [65], further supporting the use of miRNAs as predictive biomarkers for pregnancy complications.

Growing evidence implicate miRNAs in the pathogenesis of GDM [47] and suggest that maternal miRNA expression may be used as biomarkers to predict GDM. Indeed, many GDM associated miRNAs are also expressed in placentas of women with Type 1 diabetes and T2D, confirming that miRNAs expressed during GDM play an important role in metabolic regulation and reflects some of the shared aetiology between these different types of diabetes [66]. Interestingly, a subset of miRNAs were distinct for each type of diabetes, illustrating their potential to differentiate between GDM and other manifestations of diabetes. Several other studies have reported that placental miRNA expression is altered in women with GDM. Zhao et al. reported that miR-518d is upregulated in placentas of women with GDM compared to controls, and further showed that increased expression of miR-518d correlated with decreased protein expression of peroxisome proliferator-activated receptor-α (PPARα) [67], a major regulatory transcription factor in lipid homeostasis and energy metabolism [68, 69]. Li et al. identified nine miRNAs that are dysregulated in placentas of women with GDM, the expression of miR-508 was increased and miR-9, miR-27a, miR-30d, miR-33a, miR-92a, miR-137, miR-362 and miR-502 were decreased. Importantly, the decreased expression of these miRNAs correlated with increased protein expression of their gene targets, epidermal growth factor receptor (EGFR), phosphoinositide 3-Kinase (PI3K) and protein kinase B (Akt), key proteins in placental development and foetal growth [70]. Other studies showed that miR-98 [71] and miR-503 [72] are upregulated and miR-143 is downregulated [73] in placentas of women with GDM compared to women with normoglycaemic pregnancies. Intriguingly, the expression of miR-143 differentiated between GDM managed by diet or medication [71], further supporting the clinical value of miRNAs.

Xu et al. showed that the increased expression of miR-503 in the placentas of women with GDM compared to normoglycaemic pregnancies, are reflected in plasma [72]. The studies that have quantified circulating miRNA expression during GDM are summarised in **Table 1**. In 2011, Zhao et al. were the first to profile the expression of serum miRNAs during GDM [74]. Using Taqman low density arrays, followed by confirmation with individual qRT-PCR, they found that serum expression of miR-29a, miR-132 and miR-222 were decreased during GDM. Importantly, these results were validated in an internal and external cohort. Notably, serum for miRNA profiling in the discovery cohort was collected at 16–19 weeks of pregnancy, while GDM was diagnosed at 24–28 weeks of pregnancy, thus illustrating

GDM/ controls	Bio logical source	Detection method	Up-regulated	Down-regulated	No change	Normali sation	Ref
24/24* (16–19 weeks gestation)	Serum	Taqman low density array qRT-PCR	–	miR-29a miR-132 miR-222	–	Cel-miR-39	[74]
28/53 (13–31 weeks gestation)	Serum	qRT-PCR	–	miR-20a miR-222	miR-16 miR-17 miR-19a miR-19b miR-29a miR-132	Cel-miR-39	[75]
13/9 (23–31 weeks gestation)	Plasma	qRT-PCR	let-7e let-7 g miR-100 miR-101 miR-146a miR-8a miR-195 miR-222 miR-23b miR-30b miR-30c miR-30d miR-342 miR-423 miR-92a	–	–	Cel-miR-39	[76]
36/80 (7–23 weeks gestation)	Plasma	qRT-PCR	miR-155 miR-21		miR-146b miR-517 miR-222 miR-210 miR-518a miR-29a miR-223 miR-126	Cel-miR-39 and miR-423	[77]
10/10 (16–19 weeks gestation)	Plasma	Sequencing qRT-PCR	miR-16 miR-17 miR-19a miR-19b miR-20a	–	–	miR-221	[78]
85 GDM and 72 controls (16–20, 20–24 and 24–28 weeks gestation)	Plasma	qRT-PCR	miR-16 miR-17 miR-20a	–	miR-19a miR-19b	RNU6	[79]
21/10 (24–33 weeks gestation)	Plasma	qRT-PCR	miR-330	–	miR-548c	miR-374 miR-320	[92]
30/30 (24–32 weeks gestation)	Whole blood	Sequencing qRT-PCR	miR-340	–	–	RNU6B	[93]
20/20 NK	Whole blood	qRT-PCR	–	miR-494	–	RNU6	[94]

GDM/ controls	Bio logical source	Detection method	Up-regulated	Down-regulated	No change	Normali sation	Ref
67/74 (16–20, 20–24 and 24–28)	Serum	qRT-PCR	miR-183 miR-200b miR-125b miR-1290	–	–	Cel-miR-39	[95]
11/12 (third trimester)	Plasma	qRT-PCR	miR-137	–	–	RNU6	[81]
25/25 NK	Plasma	qRT-PCR	miR-503	–	–	NK	[72]

Validated in internal (36 GDM/36 controls) and two external cohorts (16 GDM/16 controls each).
GDM: gestational diabetes mellitus; qRT-PCR: quantitative real time polymerase chain reaction; NK: not known.

Table 1.
Studies investigating microRNA expression in maternal blood during gestational diabetes mellitus.

the potential of these miRNAs as screening tools for GDM. Recently, Pheiffer et al. reported that the expression of miR-29a, miR-132 and miR-222 were similarly decreased in the serum of South African women with GDM, however, only the latter was statistically significant [75]. Conflictingly, Tagoma et al. showed that miR-222 was increased in plasma of women with GDM compared to normoglycaemic pregnancies [76]. Moreover, Wander et al., observed no differences in the expression of miR-29a and miR-222 in the plasma of American women with or without GDM [77], thus illustrating the heterogeneity of miRNA expression.

In 2015, Zhu et al. used high-throughput sequencing and qRT-PCR to investigate miRNAs in plasma samples of Chinese women with or without GDM [78]. Five miRNAs (miR-16, miR-17, miR-19a, miR-19b and miR-20a) were significantly upregulated in women with GDM compared to controls. Furthermore, the differential expression of these miRNAs were observed at 16–19 weeks of pregnancy, before GDM diagnosis, once again illustrating the diagnostic value of miRNAs [78]. Cao et al. similarly demonstrated increased expression of plasma miR-16, miR-17 and miR-20a in a larger cohort of Chinese women, however, they did not observe differences in the expression of miR-19a and miR-19b [79]. More recently, Pheiffer et al. reported conflicting results. The expression of all five miRNAs were decreased in South African women with GDM, however, only the decreased expression of miR-20a was statistically significant [75]. Interestingly, regression analysis showed that miR-20a was a significant predictor of GDM, while age and body mass index were not.

Although these miRNAs were identified in plasma or serum, bioinformatics [75, 78] and experimental [74] functional analyses provided support for their biological relevance and role in the pathogenesis of GDM. Other studies also confirm the importance of miRNAs during GDM. For example, in 2014, Shi et al. reported that the expression of miR-222 is increased in omental tissue from women with GDM compared to women with normoglycaemic pregnancies, and conducted elegant *in vitro* experiments to demonstrate that miR-222 potentially regulates oestrogen-induced insulin resistance during GDM. As shown in **Table 1**, many more miRNAs have been reported to exhibit altered expression in maternal blood during GDM, however, these were investigated in single studies only.

6. Gestational diabetes and foetal microRNA expression

Dysregulated miRNA expression has been reported in human umbilical vein endothelial cells (HUVECs) of foetuses exposed to GDM. Floris et al. reported that impaired HUVEC function during GDM is associated with altered miR-101 expression [80]. Several other miRNAs, miR-137 [81], miR-let-7a, miR-let-7g, miR-30c, miR-126, miR-130b, miR-148a and miR-452 [82] were upregulated in HUVECs from infants born to mothers with GDM, suggesting that miRNAs reflect the adverse *in utero* environment imposed by GDM. Tryggestad et al. further showed that two of these miRNAs, miR-130b and miR-148a, target and decrease the expression of 5′ Adenosine monophosphate-activated protein kinase (AMPKα1), whose protein expression is decreased in placenta exposed to GDM [82]. Recently, altered miRNA expression in offspring blood was shown to be associated with birth weight [83]. MiR-33b and miR-375 were overexpressed during macrosomia, while miR-454 was overexpressed in blood of both low birth weight and macrosomic compared to normal birth weight offspring [83]. Aberrant miR-346 and miR-582 expression in cord blood were shown to be associated with foetal complications [54]. Taken together, these studies provide evidence that GDM induces dysregulated miRNA expression in offspring, which may predispose them to metabolic disease in later life. Thus, miRNAs offer potential to predict disease in offspring, which could facilitate intervention strategies to prevent future disease.

7. Challenges of microRNA profiling

Despite their stability and relative ease of quantification, analysis of circulating miRNAs present several pre-analytical and analytical challenges [84] that must be addressed before they can be used clinically. Many studies have reported that miRNA expression is affected by sample type, method of miRNA extraction, and quantification and data normalisation strategies. Differences in miRNA expression between whole blood and serum [42], between different cell types in whole blood [85, 86], between plasma and serum [87, 88] and between placenta, plasma and cord blood [54] have been described. Furthermore, miRNA expression varies according to the extraction kit used [88]. Currently, qRT-PCR is considered the gold standard for miRNA analysis, however variations between qRT-PCR platforms [87] and between qRT-PCR and other measurement platforms [22, 42, 87, 88] have been widely reported. Furthermore, data normalisation is a significant challenge during miRNA profiling, particularly extracellular miRNAs [89]. Currently, there is no consensus on the best normalisation strategy to use when profiling circulating miRNAs, although strategies based on exogenous spike-in-controls such as *C. elegans* miR-39 have been shown to be less variable than using endogenous miRNAs [88]. Moreover, heterogeneous miRNA expression is observed between populations, mediated by both genetic and environmental factors [90, 91]. During pregnancy, gestation time is also reported to affect miRNA expression [55]. Lastly, miRNAs are non-specific. For example, a single miRNA can regulate up to 200 different genes [27, 28], thus miRNAs found to be associated with GDM, may possibly be involved in other conditions as well.

8. Perspectives and recommendations for future research

MiRNAs offer great potential as biomarkers for GDM. However, they face many challenges that need to be addressed before they can become clinically applicable. Standardisation of pre-analytical and analytical methods for miRNA research may minimise the lack of reproducibility between studies and should be prioritised in miRNA research [22]. MiRNAs are epigenetic mechanisms that are regulated by various factors [90, 91], which need to be considered in miRNA studies. Large prospective cohort studies should be conducted to elucidate how biological, genetic and environmental factors affect miRNA expression, and to identify plausible diagnostic or prognostic candidates. Moreover, due to their non-specificity [27, 28], it is recommended that a panel of miRNAs, either alone, or in combination with other risk factors, should be used to increase the specificity of risk stratification models for GDM.

9. Conclusions

In this review the current status of miRNAs as biomarkers for GDM was discussed, together with recommendations for research. We provide evidence to show that miRNAs possess tremendous potential as routine screening tools, which could facilitate earlier diagnosis and management of GDM with dietary modifications or therapeutic intervention. A growing number of studies have demonstrated their clinical utility, and technological advances can lead to the development of inexpensive, point-of-care miRNA diagnostic tests in the future. However, at present miRNA profiling during GDM remains inconclusive, largely due to the irreproducibility of results between studies. Many technical, analytical and biological challenges hamper miRNA research, and must be addressed before these small RNA molecules, which are master regulators of gene expression, can become clinically applicable.

Acknowledgements

This work was funded by the South African Medical Research Council.

Conflict of interest

The authors have no conflict of interest to declare.

Author details

Carmen Pheiffer[1,2]*, Stephanie Dias[1,3], Paul Rheeder[4] and Sumaiya Adam[3]

1 Biomedical Research and Innovation Platform, South African Medical Research Council, Tygerberg, South Africa

2 Division of Medical Physiology, Faculty of Medicine and Health Sciences, University of Stellenbosch, Tygerberg, South Africa

3 Department of Obstetrics and Gynaecology, University of Pretoria, Pretoria, South Africa

4 Department of Internal Medicine, University of Pretoria, Pretoria, South Africa

*Address all correspondence to: carmen.pheiffer@mrc.ac.za

References

[1] Ferrara A. Increasing prevalence of gestational diabetes mellitus. Diabetes Care. 2007;**30**:S141-S146. DOI: 10.2337/dc07-s206

[2] International Diabetes Federation. IDF Diabetes Atlas. 8th ed. Brussels, Belgium: International Diabetes Federation; 2017. http://www.diabetesatlas.org

[3] Agarwal MM. Gestational diabetes mellitus: Screening with fasting plasma glucose. World Journal of Diabetes. 2016;**7**:279-289. DOI: 10.4239/wjd.v7.i14.279

[4] Bellamy L, Casas J-P, Hingorani AD, Williams D. Type 2 diabetes mellitus after gestational diabetes: A systematic review and meta-analysis. Lancet. 2009;**373**:1773-1779. DOI: 10.1016/S0140-6736(09)60731-5

[5] Mitanchez D, Yzydorczyk C, Siddeek B, Boubred F, Benahmed M, Simeoni U. The offspring of the diabetic mother—Short- and long-term implications. Best Practice & Research. Clinical Obstetrics & Gynaecology. 2015;**29**:256-269. DOI: 10.1016/j.bpobgyn.2014.08.004

[6] Ratner RE. Prevention of type 2 diabetes in women with previous gestational diabetes. Diabetes Care. 2007;**30**:S242-S245. DOI: 10.2337/dc07-s223

[7] Falavigna M, Schmidt MI, Trujillo J, Alves LF, Wendland ER, Torloni MR, et al. Effectiveness of gestational diabetes treatment: A systematic review with quality of evidence assessment. Diabetes Research and Clinical Practice. 2012;**98**:396-405. DOI: 10.1016/j.diabres.2012.09.002

[8] Duran A, Sáenz S, Torrejón MJ, Bordiú E, Del Valle L, Galindo M, et al. Introduction of IADPSG criteria for the screening and diagnosis of gestational diabetes mellitus results in improved pregnancy outcomes at a lower cost in a large cohort of pregnant women: The St. Carlos Gestational Diabetes Study. Diabetes Care. 2014;**37**:2442-2450. DOI: 10.2337/dc14-0179

[9] Hernandez TL, Van Pelt RE, Anderson MA, Daniels LJ, West NA, Donahoo WT, et al. A higher-complex carbohydrate diet in gestational diabetes mellitus achieves glucose targets and lowers postprandial lipids: A randomized crossover study. Diabetes Care. 2014;**37**:1254-1262. DOI: 10.2337/dc13-2411

[10] Kelley KW, Carroll DG, Meyer A. A review of current treatment strategies for gestational diabetes mellitus. Drugs in Context. 2015;**4**:212282. DOI: 10.7573/dic.212282

[11] Santangelo C, Zicari A, Mandosi E, Scazzocchio B, Mari E, Morano S, et al. Could gestational diabetes mellitus be managed through dietary bioactive compounds? Current knowledge and future perspectives. British Journal of Nutrition. 2016;**115**:1129-1144. DOI: 10.1017/S0007114516000222

[12] World Health Organization. Definition, Diagnosis and Classification of Diabetes Mellitus and its Complications. Geneva: World Health Organization; 1999

[13] Xu Y, Shen S, Sun L, Yang H, Jin B, Cao X. Metabolic syndrome risk after gestational diabetes: A systematic review and meta-analysis. PLoS One. 2014;**9**:e87863. DOI: 10.1371/journal.pone.0087863

[14] Li J-W, He S-Y, Liu P, Luo L, Zhao L, Xiao Y-B. Association of gestational diabetes mellitus (GDM) with subclinical atherosclerosis: A systemic review and meta-analysis. BMC

Cardiovascular Disorders. 2014;**14**:132. DOI: 10.1186/1471-2261-14-132

[15] Park YM, O'Brien KM, Zhao S, Weinberg CR, Baird DD, Sandler DP. Gestational diabetes mellitus may be associated with increased risk of breast cancer. British Journal of Cancer. 2017;**116**:960-963. DOI: 10.1038/bjc.2017.34

[16] Silveira PP, Portella AK, Goldani MZ, Barbieri MA. Developmental origins of health and disease (DOHaD). The Journal of Pediatrics. 2007;**83**:494-504. DOI: 10.2223/JPED.1728

[17] Barker DJ. Maternal nutrition, fetal nutrition, and disease in later life. Nutrition. 1997;**13**:807-813

[18] Chu SY, Callaghan WM, Kim SY, Schmid CH, Lau J, England LJ, et al. Maternal obesity and risk of gestational diabetes mellitus. Diabetes Care. 2007;**30**:2070-2076. DOI: 10.2337/dc06-2559a

[19] Adam S, Pheiffer C, Dias S, Rheeder P. Association between gestational diabetes and biomarkers: A role in diagnosis. Biomarkers. 2018;**23**:386-391. DOI: 10.1080/1354750X.2018.1432690

[20] Cosson E, Benbara A, Pharisien I, Nguyen MT, Revaux A, Lormeau B, et al. Diagnostic and prognostic performances over 9 years of a selective screening strategy for gestational diabetes mellitus in a cohort of 18,775 subjects. Diabetes Care. 2013;**36**:598-603. DOI: 10.2337/dc12-1428

[21] Hulka B. Overview of biological markers. In: Hulka BS, Griffith JD, Wilcosky TC, editors. Biological Markers in Epidemiology. New York: Oxford University Press; 1990. pp. 3-15

[22] Etheridge A, Lee I, Hood L, Galas D, Wang K. Extracellular microRNA: A new source of biomarkers. Mutation Research. 2011;**717**:85-90. DOI: 10.1016/j.mrfmmm.2011.03.004

[23] Guay C, Roggli E, Nesca V, Jacovetti C, Regazzi R. Diabetes mellitus, a microRNA-related disease? Translational Research. 2011;**157**:253-264. DOI: 10.1016/j.trsl.2011.01.009

[24] Lee RC, Feinbaum RL, Ambros V. The *C. elegans* heterochronic gene lin-4 encodes small RNAs with antisense complementarity to lin-14. Cell. 1993;**75**:843-854

[25] Bartel DP. MicroRNAs: Genomics, biogenesis, mechanism, and function. Cell. 2004;**116**:281-297

[26] Guo H, Ingolia NT, Weissman JS, Bartel DP. Mammalian microRNAs predominantly act to decrease target mRNA levels. Nature. 2010;**466**:835-840. DOI: 10.1038/nature09267

[27] Krek A, Grün D, Poy MN, Wolf R, Rosenberg L, Epstein EJ, et al. Combinatorial microRNA target predictions. Nature Genetics. 2005;**37**:495-500. DOI: 10.1038/ng1536

[28] Lewis BP, Burge CB, Bartel DP. Conserved seed pairing, often flanked by adenosines, indicates that thousands of human genes are microRNA targets. Cell. 2005;**120**:15-20. DOI: 10.1016/j.cell.2004.12.035

[29] Friedman RC, Farh KK-H, Burge CB, Bartel DP. Most mammalian mRNAs are conserved targets of microRNAs. Genome Research. 2009;**19**:92-105. DOI: 10.1101/gr.082701.108

[30] Ardekani AM, Naeini MM. The role of MicroRNAs in human diseases. Avicenna Journal of Medical Biotechnology. 2010;**2**:161-179

[31] Regazzi R. MicroRNAs as therapeutic targets for the treatment of diabetes mellitus and its complications. Expert Opinion on Therapeutic

Targets. 2018;**22**:153-160. DOI: 10.1080/14728222.2018.1420168

[32] Creemers EE, Tijsen AJ, Pinto YM. Circulating microRNAs: Novel biomarkers and extracellular communicators in cardiovascular disease? Circulation Research. 2012;**110**:483-495. DOI: 10.1161/CIRCRESAHA.111.247452

[33] Guay C, Regazzi R. Exosomes as new players in metabolic organ cross-talk. Diabetes, Obesity & Metabolism. 2017;**19**:S137-S146. DOI: 10.1111/dom.13027

[34] Turchinovich A, Weiz L, Burwinkel B. Extracellular miRNAs: The mystery of their origin and function. Trends in Biochemical Sciences. 2012;**37**:460-465. DOI: 10.1016/j.tibs.2012.08.003

[35] Guay C, Regazzi R. New emerging tasks for microRNAs in the control of β-cell activities. Biochimica et Biophysica Acta. 2016;**1861**:2121-2129. DOI: 10.1016/j.bbalip.2016.05.003

[36] Jung M, Schaefer A, Steiner I, Kempkensteffen C, Stephan C, Erbersdobler A, et al. Robust microRNA stability in degraded RNA preparations from human tissue and cell samples. Clinical Chemistry. 2010;**56**:998-1006. DOI: 10.1373/clinchem.2009.141580

[37] Pritchard CC, Cheng HH, Tewari M. MicroRNA profiling: Approaches and considerations. Nature Reviews. Genetics. 2012;**13**:358-369. DOI: 10.1038/nrg3198

[38] Mayeux R. Biomarkers: Potential uses and limitations. NeuroRx. 2004;**1**:182-188. DOI: 10.1602/neurorx.1.2.182

[39] Zampetaki A, Kiechl S, Drozdov I, Willeit P, Mayr U, Prokopi M, et al. Plasma microRNA profiling reveals loss of endothelial miR-126 and other microRNAs in type 2 diabetes. Circulation Research. 2010;**107**:810-817. DOI: 10.1161/CIRCRESAHA.110.226357

[40] Zampetaki A, Mayr M. MicroRNAs in vascular and metabolic disease. Circulation Research. 2012;**110**:508-522. DOI: 10.1161/CIRCRESAHA.111.247445

[41] Karolina DS, Armugam A, Tavintharan S, Wong MT, Lim SC, Sum CF, et al. MicroRNA 144 impairs insulin signaling by inhibiting the expression of insulin receptor substrate 1 in type 2 diabetes mellitus. PLoS One. 2011;**6**:e22839. DOI: 10.1371/journal.pone.0022839

[42] Dias HS, Muller C, Louw J, Pheiffer C. MicroRNA expression varies according to glucose tolerance, measurement platform, and biological source. BioMed Research International. 2017;**2017**:1080157. DOI: 10.1155/2017/1080157

[43] Pheiffer C, Dias S, Willmer T, Pace R, Aagaard K, Louw J. Altered microRNA expression during impaired glucose tolerance and high-fat diet feeding. Experimental and Clinical Endocrinology & Diabetes. 11 Jun 2018. DOI: 10.1055/a-0619-4576. [Epub ahead of print]

[44] Párrizas M, Brugnara L, Esteban Y, González-Franquesa A, Canivell S, Murillo S, et al. Circulating miR-192 and miR-193b are markers of prediabetes and are modulated by an exercise intervention. The Journal of Clinical Endocrinology and Metabolism. 2015;**100**:E407-E415. DOI: 10.1210/jc.2014-2574

[45] Luo M, Li R, Deng X, Ren M, Chen N, Zeng M, et al. Platelet-derived miR-103b as a novel biomarker for the early diagnosis of type 2 diabetes. Acta Diabetologica. 2015;**52**:943-949. DOI: 10.1007/s00592-015-0733-0

[46] Cai M, Kolluru GK, Ahmed A. Small molecule, big prospects:

MicroRNA in pregnancy and its complications. Journal of Pregnancy. 2017;**2017**:6972732. DOI: 10.1155/2017/6972732

[47] Poirier C, Desgagné V, Guérin R, Bouchard L. MicroRNAs in pregnancy and gestational diabetes mellitus: Emerging role in maternal metabolic regulation. Current Diabetes Reports. 2017;**17**:35. DOI: 10.1007/s11892-017-0856-5

[48] Pineles BL, Romero R, Montenegro D, Tarca AL, Han YM, Kim YM, et al. Distinct subsets of microRNAs are expressed differentially in the human placentas of patients with preeclampsia. American Journal of Obstetrics and Gynecology. 2007;**196**:261.e1-261.e6. DOI: 10.1016/j.ajog.2007.01.008

[49] Zhu X, Han T, Sargent IL, Yin G, Yao Y. Differential expression profile of microRNAs in human placentas from preeclamptic pregnancies vs normal pregnancies. American Journal of Obstetrics and Gynecology. 2009;**200**:661.e1-661.e7. DOI: 10.1016/j.ajog.2008.12.045

[50] Hu Y, Li P, Hao S, Liu L, Zhao J, Hou Y. Differential expression of microRNAs in the placentae of Chinese patients with severe pre-eclampsia. Clinical Chemistry and Laboratory Medicine. 2009;**47**:923-929. DOI: 10.1515/CCLM.2009.228

[51] Wang W, Feng L, Zhang H, Hachy S, Satohisa S, Laurent LC, et al. Preeclampsia up-regulates angiogenesis-associated MicroRNA (i.e., miR-17, -20a, and -20b) that target Ephrin-B2 and EPHB4 in human placenta. The Journal of Clinical Endocrinology and Metabolism. 2012;**97**:E1051-E1059. DOI: 10.1210/jc.2011-3131.

[52] Niu Z-R, Han T, Sun X-L, Luan L-X, Gou W-L, Zhu X-M. MicroRNA-30a-3p is overexpressed in the placentas of patients with preeclampsia and affects trophoblast invasion and apoptosis by its effects on IGF-1. American Journal of Obstetrics and Gynecology. 2018;**218**:249.e1-249.e12. DOI: 10.1016/j.ajog.2017.11.568

[53] Li J, Chen L, Tang Q, Wu W, Gu H, Liu L, et al. The role, mechanism and potentially novel biomarker of microRNA-17-92 cluster in macrosomia. Scientific Reports. 2015;**5**:17212. DOI: 10.1038/srep17212

[54] Tsai P-Y, Li S-H, Chen W-N, Tsai H-L, Su M-T. Differential miR-346 and miR-582-3p expression in association with selected maternal and fetal complications. International Journal of Molecular Sciences. 2017;**18.pii**:E1570. DOI: 10.3390/ijms18071570

[55] Chim SS, Shing TK, Hung EC, Leung T-Y, Lau T-K, Chiu RW, et al. Detection and characterization of placental microRNAs in maternal plasma. Clinical Chemistry. 2008;**54**:482-490. DOI: 10.1373/clinchem.2007.097972

[56] Luo S-S, Ishibashi O, Ishikawa G, Ishikawa T, Katayama A, Mishima T, et al. Human villous trophoblasts express and secrete placenta-specific microRNAs into maternal circulation via exosomes. Biology of Reproduction. 2009;**81**:717-729. DOI: 10.1095/biolreprod.108.075481

[57] Miura K, Morisaki S, Abe S, Higashijima A, Hasegawa Y, Miura S, et al. Circulating levels of maternal plasma cell-free pregnancy-associated placenta-specific microRNAs are associated with placental weight. Placenta. 2014;**35**:848-851. DOI: 10.1016/j.placenta.2014.06.002

[58] Hasegawa Y, Miura K, Higashijima A, Abe S, Miura S, Yoshiura K, et al. Increased levels of cell-free miR-517a and decreased levels of cell-free miR-518b in maternal plasma samples from placenta previa pregnancies at

32 weeks of gestation. Reproductive Sciences. 2015;**22**:1569-1576. DOI: 10.1177/1933719115589407

[59] Miura K, Higashijima A, Murakami Y, Fuchi N, Tsukamoto O, Abe S, et al. Circulating levels of pregnancy-associated, placenta-specific microRNAs in pregnant women with placental abruption. Reproductive Sciences. 2017;**24**:148-155. DOI: 10.1177/1933719116653837

[60] Hromadnikova I, Kotlabova K, Ondrackova M, Kestlerova A, Novotna V, Hympanova L, et al. Circulating C19MC microRNAs in preeclampsia, gestational hypertension, and fetal growth restriction. Mediators of Inflammation. 2013;**2013**:186041. DOI: 10.1155/2013/186041

[61] Hromadnikova I, Kotlabova K, Ivankova K, Krofta L. First trimester screening of circulating C19MC microRNAs and the evaluation of their potential to predict the onset of preeclampsia and IUGR. PLoS One. 2017;**12**:e0171756. DOI: 10.1371/journal.pone.0171756

[62] Jiang H, Wen Y, Hu L, Miao T, Zhang M, Dong J. Serum microRNAs as diagnostic biomarkers for macrosomia. Reproductive Sciences. 2015;**22**:664-671. DOI: 10.1177/1933719114561557

[63] Miura K, Higashijima A, Murakami Y, Tsukamoto O, Hasegawa Y, Abe S, et al. Circulating chromosome 19 miRNA cluster microRNAs in pregnant women with severe pre-eclampsia. The Journal of Obstetrics and Gynaecology Research. 2015;**41**:1526-1532. DOI: 10.1111/jog.12749

[64] Hu L, Han J, Zheng F, Ma H, Chen J, Jiang Y, et al. Early second-trimester serum microRNAs as potential biomarker for nondiabetic macrosomia. BioMed Research International. 2014;**2014**:394125. DOI: 10.1155/2014/394125

[65] Ge Q, Zhu Y, Li H, Tian F, Xie X, Bai Y. Differential expression of circulating miRNAs in maternal plasma in pregnancies with fetal macrosomia. International Journal of Molecular Medicine. 2015;**35**:81-91. DOI: 10.3892/ijmm.2014.1989

[66] Collares CV, Evangelista AF, Xavier DJ, Rassi DM, Arns T, Foss-Freitas MC, et al. Identifying common and specific microRNAs expressed in peripheral blood mononuclear cell of type 1, type 2, and gestational diabetes mellitus patients. BMC Research Notes. 2013;**6**:491. DOI: 10.1186/1756-0500-6-491

[67] Zhao C, Zhang T, Shi Z, Ding H, Ling X. MicroRNA-518d regulates PPARα protein expression in the placentas of females with gestational diabetes mellitus. Molecular Medicine Reports. 2014;**9**:2085-2090. DOI: 10.3892/mmr.2014.2058

[68] Abbott BD. Review of the expression of peroxisome proliferator-activated receptors alpha (PPAR alpha), beta (PPAR beta), and gamma (PPAR gamma) in rodent and human development. Reproductive Toxicology. 2009;**27**:246-257. DOI: 10.1016/j.reprotox.2008.10.001

[69] Pawlak M, Lefebvre P, Staels B. Molecular mechanism of PPARα action and its impact on lipid metabolism, inflammation and fibrosis in non-alcoholic fatty liver disease. Journal of Hepatology. 2015;**62**:720-733. DOI: 10.1016/j.jhep.2014.10.039

[70] Li J, Song L, Zhou L, Wu J, Sheng C, Chen H, et al. A microRNA signature in gestational diabetes mellitus associated with risk of macrosomia. Cellular Physiology and Biochemistry. 2015;**37**:243-252. DOI: 10.1159/000430349

[71] Cao J-L, Zhang L, Li J, Tian S, Lv X-D, Wang X-Q, et al. Up-regulation of miR-98 and unraveling regulatory mechanisms in gestational diabetes mellitus. Scientific Reports. 2016;**6**:32268. DOI: 10.1038/srep32268

[72] Xu K, Bian D, Hao L, Huang F, Xu M, Qin J, et al. MicroRNA-503 contribute to pancreatic beta cell dysfunction by targeting the mTOR pathway in gestational diabetes mellitus. EXCLI Journal. 2017;**16**:1177-1187. DOI: 10.17179/excli2017-738

[73] Muralimanoharan S, Maloyan A, Myatt L. Mitochondrial function and glucose metabolism in the placenta with gestational diabetes mellitus: Role of miR-143. Clinical Science. 2016;**130**:931-941. DOI: 10.1042/CS20160076

[74] Zhao C, Dong J, Jiang T, Shi Z, Yu B, Zhu Y, et al. Early second-trimester serum miRNA profiling predicts gestational diabetes mellitus. PLoS One. 2011;**6**:e23925. DOI: 10.1371/journal.pone.0023925

[75] Pheiffer C, Dias S, Rheeder P, Adam S. Decreased expression of circulating miR-20a-5p in south African women with gestational diabetes mellitus. Molecular Diagnosis & Therapy. 2018;**22**:345-352. DOI: 10.1007/s40291-018-0325-0

[76] Tagoma A, Alnek K, Kirss A, Uibo R, Haller-Kikkatalo K. MicroRNA profiling of second trimester maternal plasma shows upregulation of miR-195-5p in patients with gestational diabetes. Gene. 2018;**672**:137-142. DOI: 10.1016/j.gene.2018.06.004

[77] Wander PL, Boyko EJ, Hevner K, Parikh VJ, Tadesse MG, Sorensen TK, et al. Circulating early- and mid-pregnancy microRNAs and risk of gestational diabetes. Diabetes Research and Clinical Practice. 2017;**132**:1-9. DOI: 10.1016/j.diabres.2017.07.024

[78] Zhu Y, Tian F, Li H, Zhou Y, Lu J, Ge Q. Profiling maternal plasma microRNA expression in early pregnancy to predict gestational diabetes mellitus. International Journal of Gynaecology and Obstetrics. 2015;**130**:49-53. DOI: 10.1016/j.ijgo.2015.01.010

[79] Cao Y-L, Jia Y-J, Xing B-H, Shi D-D, Dong X-J. Plasma microRNA-16-5p, -17-5p and -20a-5p: Novel diagnostic biomarkers for gestational diabetes mellitus. The Journal of Obstetrics and Gynaecology Research. 2017;**43**:974-981. DOI: 10.1111/jog.13317

[80] Floris I, Descamps B, Vardeu A, Mitić T, Posadino AM, Shantikumar S, et al. Gestational diabetes mellitus impairs fetal endothelial cell functions through a mechanism involving microRNA-101 and histone methyltransferase enhancer of zester homolog-2. Arteriosclerosis, Thrombosis, and Vascular Biology. 2015;**35**:664-674. DOI: 10.1161/ATVBAHA.114.304730

[81] Peng H-Y, Li H-P, Li M-Q. High glucose induces dysfunction of human umbilical vein endothelial cells by upregulating miR-137 in gestational diabetes mellitus. Microvascular Research. 2018;**118**:90-100. DOI: 10.1016/j.mvr.2018.03.002

[82] Tryggestad JB, Vishwanath A, Jiang S, Mallappa A, Teague AM, Takahashi Y, et al. Influence of gestational diabetes mellitus on human umbilical vein endothelial cell miRNA. Clinical Science. 2016;**130**:1955-1967. DOI: 10.1042/CS20160305

[83] Rodil-Garcia P, Arellanes-Licea EDC, Montoya-Contreras A, Salazar-Olivo LA. Analysis of microRNA expression in newborns with differential birth weight using newborn screening cards. International Journal of Molecular Sciences. 2017;**18**(12):pii:E2552. DOI: 10.3390/ijms18122552

[84] Kroh EM, Parkin RK, Mitchell PS, Tewari M. Analysis of circulating microRNA biomarkers in plasma and serum using quantitative reverse transcription-PCR (qRT-PCR). Methods. 2010;**50**:298-301. DOI: 10.1016/j.ymeth.2010.01.032

[85] Leidinger P, Backes C, Dahmke IN, Galata V, Huwer H, Stehle I, et al. What makes a blood cell based miRNA expression pattern disease specific?–A miRNome analysis of blood cell subsets in lung cancer patients and healthy controls. Oncotarget. 2014;**5**:9484-9497. DOI: 10.18632/oncotarget.2419

[86] Leidinger P, Backes C, Meder B, Meese E, Keller A. The human miRNA repertoire of different blood compounds. BMC Genomics. 2014;**15**:474. DOI: 10.1186/1471-2164-15-474

[87] Wang K, Yuan Y, Cho J-H, McClarty S, Baxter D, Galas DJ. Comparing the microRNA spectrum between serum and plasma. PLoS One. 2012;**7**:e41561. DOI: 10.1371/journal.pone.0041561

[88] Vigneron N, Meryet-Figuière M, Guttin A, Issartel J-P, Lambert B, Briand M, et al. Towards a new standardized method for circulating miRNAs profiling in clinical studies: Interest of the exogenous normalisation to improve miRNA signature accuracy. Molecular Oncology. 2016;**10**:981-992. DOI: 10.1016/j.molonc.2016.03.005

[89] Schwarzenbach H, da Silva AM, Calin G, Pantel K. Which is the accurate data normalisation strategy for microRNA quantification? Clinical Chemistry. 2015;**61**:1333-1342. DOI: 10.1373/clinchem.2015.239459

[90] Huang RS, Gamazon ER, Ziliak D, Wen Y, Im HK, Zhang W, et al. Population differences in microRNA expression and biological implications. RNA Biology. 2011;**8**:692-701. DOI: 10.4161/rna.8.4.16029

[91] Gulyaeva LF, Kushlinskiy NE. Regulatory mechanisms of microRNA expression. Journal of Translational Medicine. 2016;**14**:143. DOI: 10.1186/s12967-016-0893-x

Chapter 7

Leptin and Gestational Diabetes Mellitus

Pilar Guadix, Antonio Pérez-Pérez, Teresa Vilariño-García, José L. Dueñas, Julieta Maymó, Cecilia Varone and Víctor Sánchez-Margalet

Abstract

Emerging research has highlighted the importance of leptin in fetal growth and development, independent of its essential role in the regulation of feeding and energy metabolism. Leptin is now considered an important signaling molecule of the reproductive system, since it regulates the production of gonadotropins, the blastocyst formation and implantation, the normal placentation, as well as the feto-placental communication. Placental leptin is an important cytokine which regulates placental functions in an autocrine or paracrine manner. Leptin seems to play a crucial role during the first stages of pregnancy as it modulates critical processes like proliferation, protein synthesis, invasion, and apoptosis in placental cells. Furthermore, deregulation of leptin levels has been correlated with the pathogenesis of various disorders associated with reproduction and gestation, including gestational diabetes mellitus (GDM). Due to the relevant incidence of the GDM and the importance of leptin, we decided to review the latest information available about leptin action in normal and GDM pregnancies to support the idea of leptin as an important factor and/or predictor of diverse disorders associated with reproduction and pregnancy.

Keywords: leptin, reproduction, placenta, GDM, microRNAs

1. Introduction

Adipose tissue acts as an endocrine organ, secreting different molecules or adipokines. A link between body weight, adipokines, and success of pregnancy has been proposed, although it is not fully understood [1]. Leptin was the first adipokine claimed to be the "missing link" between fat and reproduction [2]. Leptin is considered as a pleiotropic hormone that regulates not only body weight but also many other functions, including the normal physiology of the reproductive system [3]. Importantly, this hormone is also produced by other tissues, especially placenta [4].

Placental formation during human gestation is crucial for embryonic progress and successful pregnancy outcome, allowing metabolic exchange and producing steroids, hormones, growth factors, and cytokines that are critical for the maintenance of pregnancy [5, 6]. Trophoblast cells play an essential role in the development of placenta. These cells differentiate in two distinct types: extravillous and villous trophoblast. In the extravillous pathway, cytotrophoblasts proliferate, differentiate into an invasive phenotype, and penetrate in the maternal decidua and myometrium. Meanwhile, in the villous pathway, mononuclear cytotrophoblasts fuse to form a specialized multinuclear syncytium called syncytiotrophoblast [7]. In normal pregnancy, trophoblast invasion is a critical step in remodeling the maternal spiral arteries to adequately perfuse the developing placenta and fetus [8]. In this sense, deregulation of leptin levels has been implicated in the pathogenesis of gestational diabetes mellitus (GDM) [9].

2. Leptin and reproduction

Reproductive function depends on the energy reserves stored in the adipose tissue. The large energy needs for a hypothetical pregnancy was the original rationale to explain the disruption of reproductive function by low fat reserves. This led to the hypothesis of an endocrine signal that conveys information to the brain about the size of fat stores [10]. Thus, leptin was the first adipokine claimed to be the "missing link" between fat and reproduction [2]. Leptin modulates satiety and energy homeostasis [11, 12] but is also produced by the placenta. Thus, it was suggested that the effects of placental leptin on the mother may contribute to endocrine-mediated alterations in energy balance, such as the mobilization of maternal fat, which occurs during the second half of pregnancy [13, 14]. In addition, leptin has been found to influence several reproductive functions, including embryo development and implantation [15]. Moreover, animal models have demonstrated that leptin-deficient mice are subfertile and fertility can be restored by exogenous leptin [16]. This adipokine may therefore play a critical role in regulating both energy homeostasis and the reproductive system [17].

Leptin increments the secretion of gonadotropin hormones, by acting centrally at the hypothalamus [18]. In addition, because leptin has been shown to be influenced by steroid hormones and can stimulate LH release, leptin may act as a permissive factor in the development of puberty [19].

Leptin can also regulate ovary functions [20–23]. Thus, leptin resistance and hyperleptinemia in obesity lead to altered follicle function, whereas in conditions in which nutritional status is suboptimal, leptin deficiency results in hypothalamic-pituitary gonadal axis dysfunction [24, 25].

In addition, a significant role of leptin in embryo implantation was proposed. Leptin receptor (LEPR) is specifically expressed at the blastocyst stage [26], and it was also reported that leptin is present in conditioned media from human blastocysts, promoting embryo development, suggesting a function in the blastocyst-endometrial dialog [27].

3. Leptin and placenta

The implantation involves complex and synchronized molecular and cellular events between the implanting embryo and uterus, and these events are regulated by autocrine and paracrine factors [5]. Fetal growth depends on the ability of the placenta to supply nutrients adequate to meet fetal demand, which increases as gestation progresses. Villous cytotrophoblast is a progenitor cell population that produces daughter cells to support the expansion of the syncytium as placental surface area increases as well as the expansion of cytotrophoblast columns, which contain the cells destined to invade maternal decidua [28]. The placenta grows exponentially in the first and early second trimester, but growth has slowed down by term [29]. Therefore, placental growth, especially in early gestation, is a prerequisite of a high-capacity transport interface. In 1997, leptin was described as a new placental hormone in humans [14]. In fact, during pregnancy, circulating leptin levels are also increased due to leptin production by trophoblastic cells [30]. After delivery, leptin levels return to normal levels [31].

To alter intracellular signaling and function, leptin must bind to the receptor (LEPR) [32]. There are six different isoforms of LEPR (a–f) that are produced by alternative RNA splicing [33]. The only isoform that has a transmembrane domain that is capable of activating signal transduction pathways is LEPRb, whereas the other five short LEPR isoforms have either a truncated or no transmembrane domain and are unable to activate signaling pathways [33]. Activation of LEPRb results in an upregulation of a number of signal transduction pathways, including the Janus kinase/signal transducers and activators of the transcription pathway (JAK/STAT), as well as the mitogen-activated protein kinase (MAPK) and phosphatidylinositol 3-kinase (PI3K) pathways [34]. Research findings do indicate that there may be fetal-to-maternal leptin exchange across the placenta [35]. However, to date, it is not known which receptor is mediating this transportation.

Leptin has physiological effects on the placenta, including angiogenesis, growth, and immunomodulation [13]. Leptin is now considered an important regulator during the first stages of pregnancy, modulating proliferation, invasion, apoptosis, and protein synthesis, in placenta [36–41].

The control of cell proliferation is critical for a correct placental development, and it is finely regulated [42]. Altered rates of cytotrophoblast proliferation are associated with different pathologies; levels are enhanced with increased fetal growth (macrosomia) and diminished in fetal growth restriction [42]. Others factors in maternal circulation might coordinately stimulate proliferation, differentiation, and survival [43, 44] through the activation of multiple kinases [43–45] and phosphatases [45].

During placentation, cytotrophoblasts and syncytiotrophoblast keep a subset of cells in direct contact to the villous basement membranes. In the extravillous compartment, cell proliferation favors the invasion of the uterine stroma. Similarly, in the villous compartment, cells undergo syncytial fusion directed by specific transcription factors [46].

The role of MAPK in regulating trophoblast turnover is well documented in both human and animal systems [43, 44, 47]. Moreover, it was shown that leptin induces proliferative activity in many human cell types [48–50], mainly via MAPK activation [51]. We have demonstrated that leptin promotes proliferation of trophoblast cells by this MAPK pathway [41, 52]. We have also found that leptin dose-dependently stimulates protein synthesis by the activation of translation machinery [36, 53].

In this context, it is interesting to mention the role of Sam68, an RNA-binding protein originally identified as the substrate of Src during mitosis and a member of the signal transduction and activation of RNA metabolism (STAR) family [54, 55]. Leptin stimulates Tyr-phosphorylation of Sam68 in the trophoblast, mediating the dissociation from RNA, suggesting that leptin signaling could modulate RNA metabolism [48, 56]. Recent data indicate that microRNAs have a fundamental role in a variety of physiological and pathological processes. In this context, studies of microRNA expression have revealed that some microRNAs are abundantly expressed in the placenta [57]. However, the signature of miRNAs in the placenta has yet to be elucidated.

In placental villi, cell turnover is tightly regulated, via apoptotic cascade [49]. In normal pregnancy, apoptosis is an essential feature of placental development, and it is well stablished that trophoblast apoptosis increases with placental growth and advancing gestation [50]. Leptin prevents early and late events of apoptosis via MAPK pathway [41, 52]. The role of leptin was also studied under different stress conditions like serum deprivation, hyperthermia, and acidic stress [39, 40]. Under serum deprivation, leptin increased the anti-apoptotic BCL-2 protein expression, while it downregulated the pro-apoptotic BAX and BID proteins expression as well as caspase-3 active form and cleaved PARP-1 fragment in Swan-71 cells and placental explants. In addition, it was demonstrated that p53 and its phosphorylation in Ser-46 are downregulated by leptin suggesting that leptin plays a pivotal role for apoptotic signaling by p53 [37]. Recent studies have demonstrated that MAPK and PI3K pathways are necessary for this anti-apoptotic leptin action, and it was also demonstrated that MDM-2 expression is regulated by leptin [38]. In placental explants cultured at high temperatures (40 and 42°C) and a pH acid (<7.3), the expression of Ser-46 p53, p53AIP1, p21, and caspase-3 is increased, and, these effects are significantly attenuated by leptin, indicating that leptin is a pro-survival placental cytokine [39, 40].

4. Leptin and immune system in placenta

One of the most important placental functions is to prevent embryo rejection by the maternal immune system to enable its correct development [51]. To ensure normal pregnancy, trophoblast differentiation requires potent immunomodulatory mechanisms to prevent rejection of syncytiotrophoblast and invasive trophoblast by alloreactive lymphocytes and natural killer (NK) cells present in maternal blood and decidua [58]. Inflammatory mediators such as IL-6, IL-1β, TNFα, and prostaglandins are produced and secreted by the human placenta, and these cytokines play an important role in a number of normal and abnormal inflammatory processes, including the initiation and progression of human labor [59–61]. There are several homologies between the expression and regulation of cytokines and inflammation-related genes in the placenta and in the white adipose tissue. In this regard, leptin effects include the promotion of inflammation and the modulation of adaptive and innate immunity [56, 62, 63]. Thus, placental leptin acts as an immune modulator, regulating the generation of matrix metalloproteinases, arachidonic acid products, nitric oxide production, and T cell cytokines [61]. Interestingly, leptin expression is also regulated by IL-6, IL-1α, IL-1β, and IFN-ϒ [31, 64, 65].

It was reported that leptin stimulates IL-6 secretion in human trophoblast cells [66, 67]. In addition, TNFα release from human placenta is also stimulated by leptin, and it was demonstrated that NF-κB and PPAR-γ are important mediators of this effect [68]. Recently, we have found that leptin induces HLA-G expression in placenta. HLA-G has potent immunosuppressive effects promoting apoptosis of activated CD8+ T lymphocytes, the generation of tolerogenic antigen-presenting cells, and the prevention of NK cell-mediated cytotoxicity. These data place leptin as a placental cytokine which confers to trophoblast cells a tolerogenic phenotype to prevent immunological damage during the first steps of pregnancy [69].

Pro-inflammatory leptin actions may also have significant implications in the pathogenesis of various disorders during pregnancy, such as GDM, which is characterized by increased leptin expression. In this sense, placental leptin may contribute to the incremented circulating levels of pro-inflammatory mediators that are evident in these pregnancy diseases, whereas successful pregnancy is associated with downregulation of intrauterine pro-inflammatory cytokines [9, 70, 71].

5. Leptin and gestational diabetes mellitus

Gestational diabetes mellitus, characterized by glucose intolerance diagnosed during pregnancy, is one of the most common complications in pregnancy and affects 3–8% of all pregnancies [72, 73]. The prevalence of GDM has increased in recent decades due to increased average age of pregnant females and increased risk of obesity [74]. However, GDM is associated with numerous complications including macrosomia, neonatal metabolic disorders, respiratory distress syndrome, and neonatal death as well as a predisposition for the development of metabolic syndromes and typ. 2 diabetes [75, 76].

The placenta is thought to have a critical role in the pathogenesis of gestational diabetes mellitus, as GDM-associated complications resolve following delivery. Therefore, aberrant development and functions of the placenta, including placental overgrowth, have been implicated as important factors that contribute to GDM-associated complications [77, 78]. GDM is associated with insulin resistance, hyperinsulinemia, and hyperleptinemia, and these GDM-associated conditions disturb placental nutrient transport and fetal nutrient supply [79, 80].

It has been found that leptin and LEPR expressions are increased in placenta from GDM [9, 70], and, in fact leptin was proposed as a first-trimester biochemical predictor of GDM [81, 82]. In addition it was suggested that hyperinsulinemia may regulate placental leptin production acting as a circulating signal to control fetal homeostasis [73, 83]. Furthermore, it is thought that maternal glucose regulates cord blood leptin levels, and this could explain why newborns exposed to GDM have an increased risk of obesity [84]. Comparison of the placental gene expression profile between normal and diabetic pregnancies indicates that increased leptin synthesis in GDM is correlated with higher production of pro-inflammatory cytokines such as IL-6 and TNFα, causing a chronic inflammatory environment that enhances leptin production [85].

Our group has reported that insulin induces leptin expression in trophoblastic cells by increasing leptin promoter activity [86]. It is known that leptin and insulin share several signaling pathways, such as JAK2/STAT-3, MAPK, and PI3K. Moreover, we could demonstrate that in GDM, the basal phosphorylation of STAT-3, MAPK 1/3, and Akt is increased in the placenta, with resistance to a further stimulation with leptin or insulin in vitro, suggesting synergistic interaction between insulin and leptin signaling and action in human placenta [9].

On the other hand, GDM is associated with increased incidence of polyhydramnios, due to an increase in amniotic fluid volume, suggesting that aquaporins (AQP), such as AQP9 expression, could be altered in GDM [87, 88]. Besides, when maternal circulating glucose levels are controlled, they have normal amniotic fluid volume. AQP9 is also a transporter for glycerol and may also provide this substrate to the fetus. In this context, we have found that AQP9 mRNA and protein expressions are overexpressed in placentas from women with GDM. These data could suggest that during GDM the overexpression of AQP9, which correlates with higher leptin plasma levels, increments glycerol transport to the fetus which may help to cover the increase in energy needs that may occur during this gestational metabolic disorder [89].

Nevertheless, even though any nutritional or lifestyle intervention aimed to reduce weight produce a decrease in leptin levels, both in gestational diabetes and in general population, no therapeutic intervention, using leptin as a pharmacological target, has so far been used in the management of gestational diabetes.

6. Leptin and microRNAs

Gene expression can be regulated by short (18–22-nucleotide) noncoding RNAs, microRNAs, derived from long primary transcripts (pre-microRNAs) through sequential processing by two enzymes, Drosha and Dicer, and then incorporated into the RNA silencing complex, where they target homologous mRNAs. In mice, loss or inactivation of Dicer leads to multiple developmental defects [90, 91], and it has been demonstrated that in human placenta, cytotrophoblast proliferation is increased following Dicer [92]; however, the individual microRNAs responsible for these effects are unknown. In silico network analysis identified microRNAs (miR-145 and let-7a) that influence the expression of components of nodal signaling pathways. The large network is bridged by nodal molecules, such as mitogen-activated protein kinase (MAPK1/2), and AKT, which are recognized components of pro-mitogenic signaling pathways [20]. In fact, the role of MAPK1/2 in regulating trophoblast turnover is well documented in both human and animal systems [43, 44, 47]. In this context, we have reported an increased activation of MAPK 1/2 in response to leptin in trophoblastic cells from the human placenta. Thus, it is tempting to speculate that altered microRNAs expression influences the leptin expression and contributes to the pathogenesis of the GDM. However, the signature of microRNAs in the leptin expression in the placenta both in normal pregnancy and GDM remains to be elucidated. Therefore, it will be interesting to determine, in future studies, the combined role of these microRNAs in the leptin expression in normal placenta and in placenta from pregnancy pathology associated with altered placental growth (e.g., GDM) in order to clarify the regulation of placental growth by leptin.

7. Leptin in fetal development

Obesity is associated with significantly elevated plasma leptin concentrations due to an increase in white adipose tissue compared with healthy individuals [93]. As obesity rates are increasing rapidly in the Western world, so is increasing the number of obese women who become pregnant. Importantly, obese pregnant women have significantly elevated plasma leptin concentrations compared with nonobese pregnant women throughout pregnancy [94]. Even though no differences in placental leptin production has been shown, there is a downregulation of LEPRb expression in the placenta of obese mothers, which would cause placental leptin resistance (in addition to the central leptin resistance that occurs during normal pregnancy) that may be attempting to modulate fetal growth under high-energy conditions [95, 96]. Despite the complications associated with pregnancies in obese women, the offspring may be growth restricted, normal weight, or macrosomic. However, after birth, babies born from obese mothers are exposed to elevated leptin concentrations in the maternal milk [97], which suggests that the postnatal environment may increase infant growth and development, increasing the risk of developing a number of diseases in adulthood. Therefore, alterations in maternal-placental-fetal leptin exchange may modify the development of the fetus and contribute to the increased risk of developing disease in adulthood.

8. Conclusions

In conclusion, it could be affirmed that leptin controls reproduction depending on the energy state of the body and sufficient leptin levels are a prerequisite for the maintenance of reproductive capacity. The present review was focused in placental leptin effects during gestation, when leptin levels are increased due to leptin production by trophoblastic cells. Thus, leptin has a wide range of biological functions on trophoblast cells and a role in successful establishment of pregnancy. In this sense, leptin promotes proliferation, protein synthesis, and survival of placental cells. These actions are very important since cell proliferation and apoptotic cascades are critical for the correct placental development and function. Moreover, an important role of leptin in the regulation of immune mechanisms at the maternal interface has been suggested.

Observational studies have demonstrated that states of leptin overabundance or resistance can be associated with GDM. Moreover, it is also established that obesity may lead to deregulation in leptin function that results in maternal disease and clinical studies demonstrate an impact of obesity with an increased risk of a number of diseases in adulthood, including metabolic disease. In this context, leptin deregulation has been implicated in the pathogenesis of GDM. It is well accepted that leptin and LEPR expressions are increased in placentas from GDM, which may be relevant to control fetal homeostasis. Moreover, a role for microRNAs in the regulation of placental growth has been suggested, and expression profiling in the studies has shown expression and gestational changes in microRNA levels that demand functional evaluation. Further investigation is needed to fully elucidate the association of leptin with GDM and to stablish leptin as a biomarker for this pathology or the development of microRNA-based approaches to therapeutic targeting for correcting the abnormal placental growth and cell turnover seen in GDM.

Disclosure of interests

The authors declare no conflict of interest.

Author details

Pilar Guadix[1†], Antonio Pérez-Pérez[2†], Teresa Vilariño-García[2], José L. Dueñas[1], Julieta Maymó[3], Cecilia Varone[3] and Víctor Sánchez-Margalet[2*]

1 Obstetrics and Gynecology Unit, Virgen Macarena University Hospital, University of Seville, Spain

2 Department of Medical Biochemistry and Molecular Biology, and Immunology, Virgen Macarena University Hospital, University of Seville, Seville, Spain

3 Laboratory of Placental Molecular Physiology, Department of Biological Chemistry, School of Sciences, University of Buenos Aires, Argentina

*Address all correspondence to: margalet@us.es

†These authors contribute equally to this work as first authors

References

[1] El husseny MWA, Mamdouh M, Shaban S, Ibrahim Abushouk A, Zaki MMM, Ahmed OM, et al. Adipokines: Potential therapeutic targets for vascular dysfunction in type II diabetes mellitus and obesity. Journal Diabetes Research. 2017;**2017**:1-11. DOI: 10.1155/2017/8095926

[2] Friedman JM, Halaas JL. Leptin and the regulation of body weight in mammals. Nature. 1998;**395**:763-770. DOI: 10.1038/27376

[3] Pérez-Pérez A, Sánchez-Jiménez F, Maymó J, Dueñas JL, Varone C, Sánchez-Margalet V. Role of leptin in female reproduction. Clinical Chemistry and Laboratory Medicine. 2015;**53**:15-28. DOI: 10.1515/cclm-2014-0387

[4] Reitman ML, Bi S, Marcus-Samuels B, Gavrilova O. Leptin and its role in pregnancy and fetal development—An overview. Biochemical Society Transactions. 2001;**29**:68-72

[5] Staun-Ram E, Shalev E. Human trophoblast function during the implantation process. Reproductive Biology and Endocrinology. 2005;**3**:56. DOI: 10.1186/1477-7827-3-56

[6] Pollheimer J, Knöfler M. Signalling pathways regulating the invasive differentiation of human trophoblasts: A review. Placenta. 2005;**26**(Suppl A): S21-S30. DOI: 10.1016/j.placenta.2004.11.013

[7] Carson DD, Bagchi I, Dey SK, Enders AC, Fazleabas AT, Lessey BA, et al. Embryo implantation. Developmental Biology. 2000;**223**:217-237. DOI: 10.1006/dbio.2000.9767

[8] E Davies J, Pollheimer J, Yong HEJ, Kokkinos MI, Kalionis B, Knöfler M, et al. Epithelial-mesenchymal transition during extravillous trophoblast differentiation. Cell Adhesion & Migration. 2016;**10**:310-321. DOI: 10.1080/19336918.2016.1170258

[9] Pérez-Pérez A, Guadix P, Maymó J, Dueñas J, Varone C, Fernández-Sánchez M, et al. Insulin and leptin signaling in placenta from gestational diabetic subjects. Hormone and Metabolic Research. 2015;**48**:62-69. DOI: 10.1055/s-0035-1559722

[10] Elmquist JK. Anatomic basis of leptin action in the hypothalamus. Frontiers of Hormone Research. 2000;**26**:21-41

[11] Zhang Y, Proenca R, Maffei M, Barone M, Leopold L, Friedman JM. Positional cloning of the mouse obese gene and its human homologue. Nature. 1994;**372**:425-432. DOI: 10.1038/372425a0

[12] Houseknecht KL, Portocarrero CP. Leptin and its receptors: Regulators of whole-body energy homeostasis. Domestic Animal Endocrinology. 1998;**15**:457-475

[13] Hoggard N, Haggarty P, Thomas L, Lea RG. Leptin expression in placental and fetal tissues: Does leptin have a functional role? Biochemical Society Transactions. 2001;**29**:57-63

[14] Masuzaki H, Ogawa Y, Sagawa N, Hosoda K, Matsumoto T, Mise H, et al. Nonadipose tissue production of leptin: Leptin as a novel placenta-derived hormone in humans. Nature Medicine. 1997;**3**:1029-1033

[15] Acconcia F, Kumar R. Signaling regulation of genomic and nongenomic functions of estrogen receptors. Cancer Letters. 2006;**238**:1-14. DOI: 10.1016/j.canlet.2005.06.018

[16] González RR, Simón C, Caballero-Campo P, Norman R, Chardonnens D,

Devoto L, et al. Leptin and reproduction. Human Reproduction Update;**6**:290-300

[17] Sartori C, Lazzeroni P, Merli S, Patianna VD, Viaroli F, Cirillo F, et al. From placenta to polycystic ovarian syndrome: The role of adipokines. Mediators of Inflammation. 2016;**2016**: 4981916. DOI: 10.1155/2016/4981916

[18] Louis GW, Greenwald-Yarnell M, Phillips R, Coolen LM, Lehman MN, Myers MG. Molecular mapping of the neural pathways linking leptin to the neuroendocrine reproductive axis. Endocrinology. 2011;**152**:2302-2310. DOI: 10.1210/en.2011-0096

[19] Jin L, Zhang S, Burguera BG, Couce ME, Osamura RY, Kulig E, et al. Leptin and leptin receptor expression in rat and mouse pituitary cells. Endocrinology. 2000;**141**:333-339. DOI: 10.1210/endo.141.1.7260

[20] Archanco M, Muruzábal FJ, Llopiz D, Garayoa M, Gómez-Ambrosi J, Frühbeck G, et al. Leptin expression in the rat ovary depends on estrous cycle. The Journal of Histochemistry and Cytochemistry. 2003;**51**:1269-1277. DOI: 10.1177/002215540305101003

[21] Karlsson C, Lindell K, Svensson E, Bergh C, Lind P, Billig H, et al. Expression of functional leptin receptors in the human ovary. The Journal of Clinical Endocrinology and Metabolism. 1997;**82**:4144-4148. DOI: 10.1210/jcem.82.12.4446

[22] Cioffi JA, Van Blerkom J, Antczak M, Shafer A, Wittmer S, Snodgrass HR. The expression of leptin and its receptors in pre-ovulatory human follicles. Molecular Human Reproduction. 1997;**3**:467-472

[23] Ricci AG, Di Yorio MP, Faletti AG. Inhibitory effect of leptin on the rat ovary during the ovulatory process. Reproduction. 2006;**132**:771-780. DOI: 10.1530/rep.1.01164

[24] Sir-Petermann T, Recabarren SE, Lobos A, Maliqueo M, Wildt L. Secretory pattern of leptin and LH during lactational amenorrhoea in breastfeeding normal and polycystic ovarian syndrome women. Human Reproduction. 2001;**16**:244-249

[25] Farooqi IS, Jebb SA, Langmack G, Lawrence E, Cheetham CH, Prentice AM, et al. Effects of recombinant leptin therapy in a child with congenital leptin deficiency. The New England Journal of Medicine. 1999;**341**:879-884. DOI: 10.1056/NEJM199909163411204

[26] Cervero A, Horcajadas JA, Domínguez F, Pellicer A, Simón C. Leptin system in embryo development and implantation: A protein in search of a function. Reproductive Biomedicine Online. 2005;**10**:217-223

[27] Kawamura K, Sato N, Fukuda J, Kodama H, Kumagai J, Tanikawa H, et al. Leptin promotes the development of mouse preimplantation embryos in vitro. Endocrinology. 2002;**143**: 1922-1931. DOI: 10.1210/endo.143.5.8818

[28] Aplin JD. Implantation, trophoblast differentiation and haemochorial placentation: Mechanistic evidence in vivo and in vitro. Journal of Cell Science. 1991;**99**(Pt 4):681-692

[29] Schneider H. Ontogenic changes in the nutritive function of the placenta. Placenta. 1996;**17**:15-26

[30] Bajoria R, Sooranna SR, Ward BS, Chatterjee R. Prospective function of placental leptin at maternal-fetal interface. Placenta. 2002;**23**:103-115. DOI: 10.1053/plac.2001.0769

[31] Henson MC, Castracane VD. Leptin in pregnancy: An update. Biology of

Reproduction. 2006;**74**:218-229. DOI: 10.1095/biolreprod.105.045120

[32] Ahima RS, Prabakaran D, Mantzoros C, Qu D, Lowell B, Maratos-Flier E, et al. Role of leptin in the neuroendocrine response to fasting. Nature. 1996;**382**:250-252. DOI: 10.1038/382250a0

[33] Bjørbaek C, Uotani S, da Silva B, Flier JS. Divergent signaling capacities of the long and short isoforms of the leptin receptor. The Journal of Biological Chemistry. 1997;**272**:32686-32695

[34] Banks AS, Davis SM, Bates SH, Myers MG. Activation of downstream signals by the long form of the leptin receptor. The Journal of Biological Chemistry. 2000;**275**:14563-14572

[35] Wyrwoll CS, Mark PJ, Waddell BJ. Directional secretion and transport of leptin and expression of leptin receptor isoforms in human placental BeWo cells. Molecular and Cellular Endocrinology. 2005;**241**:73-79. DOI: 10.1016/j.mce.2005.05.003

[36] Pérez-Pérez A, Maymó J, Gambino Y, Dueñas JL, Goberna R, Varone C, et al. Leptin stimulates protein synthesis-activating translation machinery in human trophoblastic cells. Biology of Reproduction. 2009;**81**: 826-832. DOI: 10.1095/biolreprod.109.076513

[37] Toro AR, Maymó JL, Ibarbalz FM, Pérez-Pérez A, Maskin B, Faletti AG, et al. Leptin is an anti-apoptotic effector in placental cells involving p53 downregulation. PLoS One. 2014;**9**: e99187. DOI: 10.1371/journal.pone.0099187

[38] Toro AR, Pérez-Pérez A, Corrales Gutiérrez I, Sánchez-Margalet V, Varone CL. Mechanisms involved in p53 downregulation by leptin in trophoblastic cells. Placenta. 2015;**36**: 1266-1275. DOI: 10.1016/j.placenta.2015.08.017

[39] Pérez-Pérez A, Toro A, Vilariño-Garcia T, Guadix P, Maymó J, Dueñas JL, et al. Leptin protects placental cells from apoptosis induced by acidic stress. Cell and Tissue Research. 2018. DOI: 10.1007/s00441-018-2940-9

[40] Pérez-Pérez A, Toro AR, Vilarino-Garcia T, Guadix P, Maymó JL, Dueñas JL, et al. Leptin reduces apoptosis triggered by high temperature in human placental villous explants: The role of the p53 pathway. Placenta. 2016;**42**: 106-113. DOI: 10.1016/j.placenta.2016.03.009

[41] Magariños MP, Sánchez-Margalet V, Kotler M, Calvo JC, Varone CL. Leptin promotes cell proliferation and survival of trophoblastic cells. Biology of Reproduction. 2007;**76**:203-210. DOI: 10.1095/biolreprod.106.051391

[42] Genbacev O, Miller RK. Post-implantation differentiation and proliferation of cytotrophoblast cells: In vitro models—A review. Placenta. 2000;**21**(Suppl A):S45-S49

[43] Forbes K, Westwood M, Baker PN, Aplin JD. Insulin-like growth factor I and II regulate the life cycle of trophoblast in the developing human placenta. American Journal of Physiology. Cell Physiology. 2008;**294**: C1313-C1322. DOI: 10.1152/ajpcell.00035.2008

[44] Forbes K, Souquet B, Garside R, Aplin JD, Westwood M. Transforming growth factor-{beta} (TGF{beta}) receptors I/II differentially regulate TGF {beta}1 and IGF-binding protein-3 mitogenic effects in the human placenta. Endocrinology. 2010;**151**: 1723-1731. DOI: 10.1210/en.2009-0896

[45] Forbes K, West G, Garside R, Aplin JD, Westwood M. The protein-tyrosine phosphatase, SRC homology-2 domain

containing protein tyrosine phosphatase-2, is a crucial mediator of exogenous insulin-like growth factor signaling to human trophoblast. Endocrinology. 2009;**150**:4744-4754. DOI: 10.1210/en.2009-0166

[46] Huppertz B, Kadyrov M, Kingdom JCP. Apoptosis and its role in the trophoblast. American Journal of Obstetrics and Gynecology. 2006;**195**: 29-39. DOI: 10.1016/j.ajog.2005.07.039

[47] Saba-El-Leil MK, Vella FDJ, Vernay B, Voisin L, Chen L, Labrecque N, et al. An essential function of the mitogen-activated protein kinase Erk2 in mouse trophoblast development. EMBO Reports. 2003;**4**:964-968. DOI: 10.1038/sj.embor.embor939

[48] Sánchez-Jiménez F, Pérez-Pérez A, González-Yanes C, Najib S, Varone CL, Sánchez-Margalet V. Leptin receptor activation increases Sam68 tyrosine phosphorylation and expression in human trophoblastic cells. Molecular and Cellular Endocrinology. 2011;**332**: 221-227. DOI: 10.1016/j.mce.2010.10.014

[49] Heazell AEP, Lacey HA, Jones CJP, Huppertz B, Baker PN, Crocker IP. Effects of oxygen on cell turnover and expression of regulators of apoptosis in human placental trophoblast. Placenta. 2008;**29**:175-186. DOI: 10.1016/j.placenta.2007.11.002

[50] Sharp AN, Heazell AEP, Crocker IP, Mor G. Placental apoptosis in health and disease. American Journal of Reproductive Immunology. 2010;**64**: 159-169. DOI: 10.1111/j.1600-0897.2010.00837.x

[51] Maltepe E, Bakardjiev AI, Fisher SJ. The placenta: Transcriptional, epigenetic, and physiological integration during development. The Journal of Clinical Investigation. 2010;**120**: 1016-1025. DOI: 10.1172/JCI41211

[52] Pérez-Pérez A, Maymó J, Dueñas JL, Goberna R, Calvo JC, Varone C, et al. Leptin prevents apoptosis of trophoblastic cells by activation of MAPK pathway. Archives of Biochemistry and Biophysics. 2008;**477**: 390-395. DOI: 10.1016/j.abb.2008.06.015

[53] Pérez-Pérez A, Gambino Y, Maymó J, Goberna R, Fabiani F, Varone C, et al. MAPK and PI3K activities are required for leptin stimulation of protein synthesis in human trophoblastic cells. Biochemical and Biophysical Research Communications. 2010;**396**:956-960. DOI: 10.1016/j.bbrc.2010.05.031

[54] Fumagalli S, Totty NF, Hsuan JJ, Courtneidge SA. A target for Src in mitosis. Nature. 1994;**368**:871-874. DOI: 10.1038/368871a0

[55] Taylor SJ, Shalloway D. An RNA-binding protein associated with Src through its SH2 and SH3 domains in mitosis. Nature. 1994;**368**:867-871. DOI: 10.1038/368867a0

[56] Sánchez-Margalet V, Martín-Romero C, Santos-Alvarez J, Goberna R, Najib S, Gonzalez-Yanes C. Role of leptin as an immunomodulator of blood mononuclear cells: Mechanisms of action. Clinical and Experimental Immunology. 2003;**133**:11-19

[57] Kotlabova K, Doucha J, Hromadnikova I. Placental-specific microRNA in maternal circulation—Identification of appropriate pregnancy-associated microRNAs with diagnostic potential. Journal of Reproductive Immunology. 2011;**89**:185-191. DOI: 10.1016/j.jri.2011.02.006

[58] Hutter H, Hammer A, Dohr G, Hunt JS. HLA expression at the maternal-fetal interface. Developmental Immunology. 1998;**6**:197-204

[59] Lappas M, Rice GE. Phospholipase A2 isozymes in pregnancy and

parturition. Prostaglandins, Leukotrienes, and Essential Fatty Acids. 2004;**70**:87-100

[60] Rice GE. Cytokines and the initiation of parturition. Frontiers of Hormone Research. 2001;**27**:113-146

[61] Lappas M, Yee K, Permezel M, Rice GE. Release and regulation of leptin, resistin and adiponectin from human placenta, fetal membranes, and maternal adipose tissue and skeletal muscle from normal and gestational diabetes mellitus-complicated pregnancies. The Journal of Endocrinology. 2005;**186**:457-465. DOI: 10.1677/joe.1.06227

[62] Lam QLK, Lu L. Role of leptin in immunity. Cellular & Molecular Immunology. 2007;**4**:1-13

[63] Fernández-Riejos P, Najib S, Santos-Alvarez J, Martín-Romero C, Pérez-Pérez A, González-Yanes C, et al. Role of leptin in the activation of immune cells. Mediators of Inflammation. 2010; **2010**:568343. DOI: 10.1155/2010/568343

[64] Fontana VA, Sanchez M, Cebral E, Calvo JC. Interleukin-1 beta regulates metalloproteinase activity and leptin secretion in a cytotrophoblast model. Biocell. 2010;**34**:37-43

[65] Fontana VA, Sanchez M, Cebral E, Calvo JC. Interferon-gamma inhibits metalloproteinase activity and cytotrophoblast cell migration. American Journal of Reproductive Immunology. 2010;**64**:20-26. DOI: 10.1111/j.1600-0897.2010.00816.x

[66] Soh EB, Mitchell MD, Keelan JA. Does leptin exhibit cytokine-like properties in tissues of pregnancy? American Journal of Reproductive Immunology. 2000;**43**:292-298

[67] Cameo P, Bischof P, Calvo JC. Effect of leptin on progesterone, human chorionic gonadotropin, and interleukin-6 secretion by human term trophoblast cells in culture. Biology of Reproduction. 2003;**68**:472-477

[68] Lappas M, Permezel M, Georgiou HM, Rice GE. Nuclear factor kappa B regulation of proinflammatory cytokines in human gestational tissues in vitro. Biology of Reproduction. 2002; **67**:668-673

[69] Barrientos G, Toro A, Moschansky P, Cohen M, Garcia MG, Rose M, et al. Leptin promotes HLA-G expression on placental trophoblasts via the MEK/Erk and PI3K signaling pathways. Placenta. 2015;**36**:419-426. DOI: 10.1016/j.placenta.2015.01.006

[70] Pérez-Pérez A, Maymó JL, Gambino YP, Guadix P, Dueñas JL, Varone CL, et al. Activated translation signaling in placenta from pregnant women with gestational diabetes mellitus: Possible role of leptin. Hormone and Metabolic Research. 2013;**45**:436-442. DOI: 10.1055/s-0032-1333276

[71] Qiu C, Williams MA, Vadachkoria S, Frederick IO, Luthy DA. Increased maternal plasma leptin in early pregnancy and risk of gestational diabetes mellitus. Obstetrics and Gynecology. 2004;**103**:519-525. DOI: 10.1097/01.AOG.0000113621.53602.7a

[72] Barnes-Powell LL. Infants of diabetic mothers: The effects of hyperglycemia on the fetus and neonate. Neonatal Network. 2007;**26**:283-290. DOI: 10.1891/0730-0832.26.5.283

[73] Uzelac PS, Li X, Lin J, Neese LD, Lin L, Nakajima ST, et al. Dysregulation of leptin and testosterone production and their receptor expression in the human placenta with gestational diabetes mellitus. Placenta. 2010;**31**:581-588. DOI: 10.1016/j.placenta.2010.04.002

[74] Ferrara A. Increasing prevalence of gestational diabetes mellitus: A public health perspective. Diabetes Care. 2007;

30(Supp. 2):S141-S146. DOI: 10.2337/dc07-s206

[75] Lee AJ, Hiscock RJ, Wein P, Walker SP, Permezel M. Gestational diabetes mellitus: Clinical predictors and long-term risk of developing typ. 2 diabetes: A retrospective cohort study using survival analysis. Diabetes Care. 2007;**30**:878-883. DOI: 10.2337/dc06-1816

[76] Thadhani R, Powe CE, Tjoa ML, Khankin E, Ye J, Ecker J, et al. First-trimester follistatin-like-3 levels in pregnancies complicated by subsequent gestational diabetes mellitus. Diabetes Care. 2010;**33**:664-669. DOI: 10.2337/dc09-1745

[77] Ericsson A, Säljö K, Sjöstrand E, Jansson N, Prasad PD, Powell TL, et al. Brief hyperglycaemia in the early pregnant rat increases fetal weight at term by stimulating placental growth and affecting placental nutrient transport. The Journal of Physiology. 2007;**581**:1323-1332. DOI: 10.1113/jphysiol.2007.131185

[78] Taricco E, Radaelli T, Nobile de Santis MS, Cetin I. Foetal and placental weights in relation to maternal characteristics in gestational diabetes. Placenta. 2003;**24**:343-347

[79] Desoye G, Hauguel-de Mouzon S. The human placenta in gestational diabetes mellitus. The insulin and cytokine network. Diabetes Care. 2007;**30**(Supp. 2):S120-S126. DOI: 10.2337/dc07-s203

[80] Araújo JR, Keating E, Martel F. Impact of gestational diabetes mellitus in the maternal-to-fetal transport of nutrients. Current Diabetes Reports. 2015;**15**:569. DOI: 10.1007/s11892-014-0569-y

[81] Powe CE. Early pregnancy biochemical predictors of gestational diabetes mellitus. Current Diabetes Reports. 2017;**17**:12. DOI: 10.1007/s11892-017-0834-y

[82] Iciek R, Wender-Ozegowska E, Zawiejska A, Mikolajczak P, Mrozikiewicz PM, Pietryga M, et al. Placental leptin and its receptor genes expression in pregnancies complicated by typ. 1 diabetes. Journal of Physiology and Pharmacology. 2013;**64**:579-585

[83] Lepercq J, Cauzac M, Lahlou N, Timsit J, Girard J, Auwerx J, et al. Overexpression of placental leptin in diabetic pregnancy: A critical role for insulin. Diabetes. 1998;**47**:847-850

[84] Côté S, Gagné-Ouellet V, Guay SP, Allard C, Houde AA, Perron P, et al. PPARGC1α gene DNA methylation variations in human placenta mediate the link between maternal hyperglycemia and leptin levels in newborns. Clinical Epigenetics. 2016;**8**:72. DOI: 10.1186/s13148-016-0239-9

[85] Miehle K, Stepan H, Fasshauer M. Leptin, adiponectin and other adipokines in gestational diabetes mellitus and pre-eclampsia. Clinical Endocrinology. 2012;**76**:2-11. DOI: 10.1111/j.1365-2265.2011.04234.x

[86] Pérez-Pérez A, Maymó J, Gambino Y, Guadix P, Dueñas JL, Varone C, et al. Insulin enhances leptin expression in human trophoblastic cells. Biology of Reproduction. 2013;**89**:20. DOI: 10.1095/biolreprod.113.109348

[87] Bednar AD, Beardall MK, Brace RA, Cheung CY. Differential expression and regional distribution of aquaporins in amnion of normal and gestational diabetic pregnancies. Physiological Reports. 2015;**3**:e12320. DOI: 10.14814/phy2.12320

[88] Castro Parodi M, Farina M, Dietrich V, Abán C, Szpilbarg N, Zotta E, et al. Evidence for insulin-mediated control of AQP9 expression in human placenta.

Placenta. 2011;**32**:1050-1056. DOI: 10.1016/j.placenta.2011.09.022

[89] Vilariño-García T, Pérez-Pérez A, Dietrich V, Guadix P, Dueñas JL, Varone CL, et al. Leptin upregulates aquaporin 9 expression in human placenta in vitro. Gynecological Endocrinology. 2018;**34**:175-177. DOI: 10.1080/09513590.2017.1380184

[90] Bernstein E, Kim SY, Carmell MA, Murchison EP, Alcorn H, Li MZ, et al. Dicer is essential for mouse development. Nature Genetics. 2003;**35**: 215-217. DOI: 10.1038/ng1253

[91] Yang WJ, Yang DD, Na S, Sandusky GE, Zhang Q, Zhao G. Dicer is required for embryonic angiogenesis during mouse development. The Journal of Biological Chemistry. 2005;**280**: 9330-9335. DOI: 10.1074/jbc. M413394200

[92] Forbes K, Farrokhnia F, Aplin JD, Westwood M. Dicer-dependent miRNAs provide an endogenous restraint on cytotrophoblast proliferation. Placenta. 2012;**33**:581-585. DOI: 10.1016/j.placenta.2012.03.006

[93] Garibotto G, Russo R, Franceschini R, Robaudo C, Saffioti S, Sofia A, et al. Inter-organ leptin exchange in humans. Biochemical and Biophysical Research Communications. 1998;**247**:504-509. DOI: 10.1006/bbrc.1998.8819

[94] Misra VK, Straughen JK, Trudeau S. Maternal serum leptin during pregnancy and infant birth weight: The influence of maternal overweight and obesity. Obesity (Silver Spring). 2013;**21**: 1064-1069. DOI: 10.1002/oby.20128

[95] Tessier DR, Ferraro ZM, Gruslin A. Role of leptin in pregnancy: Consequences of maternal obesity. Placenta. 2013;**34**:205-211. DOI: 10.1016/j.placenta.2012.11.035

[96] Farley DM, Choi J, Dudley DJ, Li C, Jenkins SL, Myatt L, et al. Placental amino acid transport and placental leptin resistance in pregnancies complicated by maternal obesity. Placenta. 2010;**31**:718-724. DOI: 10.1016/j.placenta.2010.06.006

[97] Dundar NO, Anal O, Dundar B, Ozkan H, Caliskan S, Büyükgebiz A. Longitudinal investigation of the relationship between breast milk leptin levels and growth in breast-fed infants. Journal of Pediatric Endocrinology & Metabolism. 2005;**18**:181-187